Critical praise for
The What's Happening to My Body? Book for Girls:

"The beauty of this book is the absolutely natural way Madaras encourages the young woman to explore, understand, and accept her own special body at the same time she is learning the basic facts of female development."   —*Siecus Report*

"She tackles some of the hardest subjects with the aim of provoking discussion between mother and daughter rather than conveying her own point of view....In reading Madaras's review of the facts together, mothers and daughters may indeed become closer to one another, and more relaxed."   —*Kirkus Reviews*

"As a gynecologist, I am delighted that this book, with its lucid and direct style, has been written....It will help set the direction for young women to keep informed throughout their lives about issues affecting their lives."
—Cynthia W. Cooke, M.D., Clinical
Assistant Professor, Obstetrics and
Gynecology, University of Pennsylvania

"Poignant and enlightening...a valuable guide for any parent who is looking for a positive way to approach the subject of sexuality with any pubescent child, male or female."
—*Charlotte News Observer*

"A wonderful reading experience...a short, packed, direct yet genteel approach to sexuality."   —*Science Books and Films*

D0097482

THE WHAT'S HAPPENING TO MY BODY?

BOOK FOR GIRLS
NEW EDITION

---

*A Growing Up Guide
for Parents and Daughters*

LYNDA MADARAS
with AREA MADARAS

Drawings by Claudia Ziroli
and Jackie Aher

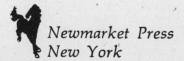

Newmarket Press
New York

91 FG 10 9 8 7 6 5 4 HC

92 93 94 95 FG 15 14 13 12   PB

Library of Congress Cataloging-in-Publication Data

Madaras, Lynda.
  The what's happening to my body? book for girls.

  Bibliography: p.
  Includes index.
  Summary: Discusses the changes that take place in a girl's body during puberty, includ-
ing information on the body's changing size and shape, pubic hair, breasts, the reproduc-
tive organs, the menstrual cycle, and puberty in boys.
    1. Adolescent girls—Growth. 2. Adolescent girls—Physiology. 3. Puberty. 4. Sex instruc-
tion for girls. [1. Sex instruction for girls. 2. Puberty. 3. Adolescent girls] I. Madaras, Area.
II. Title.
RJ144.M3 1987   613.9'55   87-28117
ISBN 1-55704-001-X
ISBN 0-937858-98-6 (pbk.)

Quantity Purchases
Companies, professional groups, clubs and other organizations may
qualify for special terms when ordering quantities of this title. For information contact: Special Sales Dept., Newmarket Press, 18 East 48th
Street, New York, New York 10017, or call (212) 832-3575.

Manufactured in the United States of America

New Edition

CONTENTS

LIST OF ILLUSTRATIONS

FOREWORD
by Cynthia W. Cooke, M.D.

The *"What's Happening to My Body?" Book for Girls* takes a uniquely positive attitude toward the subject of female puberty. Throughout the ages male puberty has been greeted as a time of celebration—the arrival of manhood. Female puberty has often been closeted in shame, as if it were not at all the same process. There are centuries of tradition—both cultural and religious—that view the menstrual period as a time of uncleanliness or sickness. This negative attitude, coupled with the general resistance to sex education in the schools, has limited the availability of accurate information for young women until now.

Puberty and adolescence can be a devisive, traumatic time for many mother-daughter relationships. Recent explosions in sexual openness and explicitness in the media have broadened the communication gap between generations. Young women are beginning sexual activity at an earlier age, and though they seem to act in a more mature fashion than previous generations, they do not usually have a deep understanding of their bodies or psyches. They often act without considering the medical or social consequences.

As a gynecologist frequently confronted with such situations, I am delighted that this book, with its lucid and direct style, has been written. It provides an important starting ground for further discussion between mothers and daughters, and it will help set the direction for young women to keep informed, throughout their lives, about issues affecting their health.

Cynthia W. Cooke, M.D.
Clinical Assistant Professor, Obstetrics
and Gynecology, University of Pennsylvania
Co-author, *The Ms. Guide to a Woman's Health*

INTRODUCTION:
Why I Wrote This Book

It was one of those perfectly languid summer days when the heat is so rich and thick you can taste the scent of summer wildflowers in the air. My eight-year-old daughter and I were slowly making our way downstream through the woods by our house. It was one of those magic moments that sometimes happen between mothers and daughters. All the years of diaper changing, complicated child-care arrangements, hectic juggling of career and motherhood, nagging about bedrooms that need cleaning and pets that need feeding, all the inevitable resentments, conflicts, and quarrels seemed to fade away, leaving just the two of us, close and connected.

We stopped to sun ourselves on a rock, and my daughter shyly told me she had some new hairs growing on her body.

"Right down there," she pointed.

I was filled with pride as I watched her scrambling among the rocks, a young colt, long-limbed and elegant and very beautiful. I marveled at her assurance and ease. Her transition into womanhood would be so much more graceful than my own halting, jerky, and sometimes painful progress through puberty.

I was also proud of our relationship, proud that she felt comfortable enough to confide in me. Never in my wildest imaginings would I have thought of telling my mother that I'd discovered pubic hairs growing on my body. It was simply not something we could have discussed. I was glad that it was going to be different between my daughter and me.

We didn't talk much more about her discovery that day. Weeks and months passed without further mention of the topic, but our relationship remained close and easy.

"Enjoy it while you can," my friends with older daughters would tell me, "because once they hit puberty, it's all over. That's when they really get an attitude. There's just no talking to them." I listened in smug silence. I knew the stereotype: the sullen, sulky adolescent daughter and the nagging harpy of a mother who can't communicate with each other; but it was going to be different for us.

My daughter must have been nine or ten when it first started— her introduction to the nasty world of playground politics and the cruel games young girls play with each other. She'd arrive home from school in tears; her former best friend was now someone else's closest ally; she'd been excluded from the up- coming slumber party or was the victim of some other calculated schoolgirl snub. She'd cry her eyes out. I didn't know what to say.

"Well, if they're going to be like that, find someone else to play with," I'd say.

The tears flowed on. It got to be a weekly, then a twice-weekly event. It went on for months and months. And then I finally began to realize that no sooner than she had dried her tears, I would hear her on the telephone, maliciously gossiping about some other little girl, a former friend, and cementing a new friendship by plotting to exclude this other girl. I was indignant, and I began to point out the inconsistency in her behavior.

"You don't understand," she'd yell, stomping off to her bed- room and slamming the door.

She was right, I didn't understand. From time to time, I'd talk to the other mothers. It was the same with all of us. Why were our daughters acting like this? None of us had any answers.

"Well, girls will be girls," sighed one mother philosophically. "They all do it and we did the same when we were their age."

I reached back over the years, trying to remember. Were we really that horrible? Then I remembered The Powder Puffs, a club my girl friends and I belonged to. Unlike the Girl Scouts and the other adult-sanctioned after-school clubs, The Powder Puffs had no formal meetings, no ostensible purpose, which is not to say that the club didn't have a purpose. It did. The membership cards, which were wondrously official looking since one girl's father had run them off in his print shop, and which we carried around in the cloudy cellophane inserts of our identi- cal vinyl, genuine leather wallets, certified us as members of the all-important Group. As if that weren't identification enough, we moved around in an inseparable herd, ate lunch together in our special territory of the playground, sat together giggling like a gaggle of geese in school assemblies, wrote each other's names on the canvas of our scuffed tennis shoes, combed our hair the same way, dressed alike, and generally made life miserable for the girls who were not members of our group.

Today, some twenty years later, I can only vaguely recall the names and faces of the other members of The Powder Puffs. I do, however, remember one girl so vividly that I can almost count the freckles on her face. Her name was Pam, and she was most emphatically not a member of the group, although she wanted desperately to be—so desperately, in fact, that she took to writing notes that she'd leave in my desk:

Dear Lynda,
  Please, Please, Please let me join The Powder Puffs. If you say I'm OK, the rest of the girls will too. Please!!! Please!!!! Please!!!!! Please, please, please!
                                                            Pam

The notes embarrassed me horribly and, of course, the mere act of writing them doomed Pam forever to the status of outsider. I have conveniently forgotten how Pam fared after that. I know she never got to be a Powder Puff, and I imagine we made her life even more miserable with snickers and snubs, behind-the-back whisperings and the usual sorts of adolescent tactics. (I wonder if it would have been any comfort to Pam to have known that a year later, when my family moved to another state, I got my comeuppance. In the vulnerable position of "the new girl," I was the perfect target and boarded the school bus each day, pretending to be oblivious to the snickers and whispers that followed me up the aisle while I hunted for a seat.)

At any rate, what's really frightening is that I wasn't any more cruel than most adolescent girls. I talk to other women about their relationships with other girls during those years and hear the same sorts of stories. The milk of human kindness does not flow freely in the veins of pubescent girls.

We all remember how it was, and it was much the same for all of us. We had our best friend, from whom we were inseparable, with whom we shared our deepest secrets, and to whom we swore everlasting friendship. And then there was the larger gang, the other little girls at school. Everyone had a role: leader, follower, victim. Although the role assignments shifted from time to time, the roles themselves remained constant.

The games we played with each other were standardized as well and not very pretty. Exclusion was the basic format. One girl, for the crime of being the smartest, the prettiest, the ugliest, the dumbest, the most sexually developed, or whatever, was designated the victim. She was cast out, ostracized by the group.

But what was even more important, what was, in fact the central theme of my life in those years was a more personalized version of the exclusion game: betrayal by the best friend. In this case, the formerly inseparable friend was now unavailable for after-school activities, Saturday afternoon movies, and so forth. Her time was taken up with the new best friend. We were abandoned, crushed, and heartbroken; we cried our eyes out.

Little boys don't spend their energies in such melodramatic psychodramas. There's the gang or, more likely, the team, even the best friend and, undoubtedly, lots of exclusion, especially for the unathletic, quiet, and gentler boys, but there is not the same intensity in their interpersonal relationships nor the petty and vicious aspects that characterize the relationships between girls of this age.

Maybe, I thought, the mother who sighed that business about "girls being girls" was right. We all did it, and now it was happening all over again. Our daughters were playing the same games, by the same rules. Maybe it was inevitable. Maybe it was just the nature of the beast. I didn't like this idea, but there it was.

To add to the things I didn't like, there was a growing tension between my daughter and me. She was terribly moody, and it seemed as if she was always angry with me. And I was often angry with her. Of course, we'd always quarreled, but now the quarrels were almost constant. The volume of our communications reached a new decibel level. There was an ever-present strain between us.

All of this bothered me a great deal, but what was even more disturbing was the change in her attitude about her body. In contrast to the shy wonder that greeted her first pubic hairs, there was now a complete horror at the idea of developing breasts and having her first period. Like most "modern" mothers, I wanted my daughter's transition from childhood to womanhood to be a comfortable, even joyous, time. I had intended to provide her with all the necessary information in a frank, straight-forward manner. This, or so went my reasoning, would eliminate any problems.

But, here was my daughter telling me she didn't want to grow breasts or have her first period. I asked why, but didn't get much further than "because I donwanna." I countered with an it's-great-to-grow-up pep talk that rang hollow even to my own ears.

Clearly something was amiss. I thought I'd made all the necessary information available in the most thoroughly modern manner, but the anticipated results, a healthy and positive attitude toward her body, had not materialized.

I thought long and hard about all of this, and finally I began to realize that I hadn't given my daughter all the information I thought I had. Although she was amazingly well informed about the most minute details of ovum and sperm, pregnancy and birth, the physical details of intercourse, and even the emotional content of love-making, she knew nothing, or next to nothing, about menstruation and the changes that would take place in her body over the next few years. She'd seen me in the bathroom changing a tampon, and I'd tossed off a quick explanation of menstrual periods, but I'd never really sat down and discussed the topic with her. I'd read her any number of marvelous children's books that explain conception, birth, and sexuality, but I'd never read her one about menstruation. Obviously, it was time to do that.

So, full of purpose, I trotted off to the library and discovered that there was no such book.* There were one or two books for young girls that briefly mentioned the topic, but they were hopelessly out of date, and the tone was all wrong. Some of them even made menstruation sound like a disease.

The more deeply I researched the topic, the less surprised I was that there was no book for young girls on menstruation. Throughout history, in culture after culture, menstruation has

---

* Since that time, some excellent books have come out. See "For Further Reading" in the back of this book.

been a taboo subject. The taboo has taken many forms: One must not eat the food cooked by a menstruating woman; touch objects she has touched; look into her eyes; have sex with her. We no longer believe that the glance of a menstruating woman will wither a field of crops, that her touch will poison the water in the well, that having sex with her will make a man's penis fall off, but the menstrual taboo is, nonetheless, alive and well.

Of course, we are no longer banished to menstrual huts each month, as were our ancestral mothers in more primitive societies. But as Nancy Friday argues in *My Mother, My Self*, our release from monthly exile does not necessarily represent a more enlightened view of menstruation. Rather, Friday says, thanks to centuries of conditioning, we have so completely internalized the menstrual taboo that it's simply no necessary to bother any longer with menstrual huts. Our modern tribe needn't go to such lengths to remove any disturbing sight or mention of menstruation from its collective consciousness. We do it ourselves, through our ladylike avoidance of any public discussion of the topic and our meticulous toilet-paper mummification of our bloodied pads and tampons.

So total is our silence that we ourselves are sometimes not aware of it.

"Oh, yes," the mother says, "I told my daughter all about it."

"My mother never told me anything," the daughter says.

Even if we are conscious of this silence and decide that it is time that this deplorable situation was dealt with, the taboos and our cultural embarrassment about menstruation may still take their toll. Wanting our daughters to have a positive view of their natural bodily functions, particularly if we have suffered in this area, we summon up our courage and carefully rehearse the proper lines. Intent upon improving the script our mothers wrote for us, we boldly announce to our daughters: "Menstruation Is a Wonderful Part of Being a Woman, a Unique Ability of Which You Should Be Proud."

At the same time, none of us would think of hiding our toothbrushes under the sink or in the back corners of the bathroom cupboard, yet it is rare to find a box of sanitary napkins prominently displayed next to the deodorants, toothpastes, and hair sprays that line the bathroom shelves of most homes. Thus, we constantly contradict our brave words and send our daughters double messages. We say it's fine and wonderful, but our unconscious actions indicate just the opposite. And, as we all know, actions speak louder than words.

The sad truth is that most of us have very little in the way of positive images to offer our daughters. Indeed, most of us are remarkably ignorant of even the basic facts about our bodies and our menstrual cycle.

As a result of the research I was doing, I was learning quite a bit about the physiological processes of menstruation. I could at least give a coherent explanation to a sixth grader, but I was also learning that I had a whole host of negative attitudes about menstruation in the back of my mind, attitudes that I had not even been conscious of before. These attitudes were changing, but who knew what else might be still lurking in the dark corridors of my subconscious? If I talked to my daughter about menstruation, I could say the right words, but would my body language, my tone of voice (and all those other unconscious ways of communicating) betray my intended message?

I worried about all of this for entirely too long a time, until the obvious solution sneaked up on me: I simply explained to my daughter that, when I was growing up, people thought of menstruation as something unclean and unmentionable. Now that I was older and more grown up, my attitudes were changing. But some of the feelings I had were old ones that I had lived with for a long time, all my life in fact, and they were hard to shake off. Sometimes they still got in my way without my even knowing it. This, of course, made perfect sense to my daughter, and from this starting point, we began to learn about our bodies together.

We didn't sit down and have The Talk. My mother sat me down one day to have The Talk, and I suppose she must have explained things in a comprehensive way, but all I remember was my mother being horribly nervous and saying a lot of things about babies and blood and that when It happened to me, I could go to the bottom drawer of her dresser and get some napkins. I wondered why she was keeping the napkins in a dresser drawer instead of in the kitchen cabinet where she usually kept them, but it didn't seem like a good time to ask questions.

Having one purposeful, nervous discussion didn't seem like

it would fill the bill. Puberty is a complicated topic and it takes more than one talk. I decided just to keep the topic in mind and bring it up now and again. It turned out to be a pretty natural thing to do since I was doing so much research on the female body. In one of the medical texts I was plodding through, there was a section on puberty that discussed the five stages of pubic hair and breast development, complete with photos. I read the section to my daughter, translating from medicalese into English, so she would know when and how these changes would happen in her body.

I talked to her about what I was learning about the workings of the menstrual cycle. I showed her some magnificent pictures taken inside a woman's body at the very moment of ovulation as the delicate, fingerlike projections on the end of the fallopian tubes were reaching out to grasp the ripe egg.

A friend's mother gave us a wonderful collection of booklets from a sanitary napkin manufacturer that dated back over a period of thirty years. We read them together, laughing at the old-fashioned attitudes, attitudes I'd grown up with.

In the course of our reading, we learned that most girls begin to have a slight vaginal discharge a year or two prior to menstruation. I had told my daughter that when she started to menstruate, I would give her the opal ring that I always wore on my left hand, and that she, in turn, could pass it on to her daughter one day. But when she discovered the first signs of vaginal discharge, we were both so elated that I gave her the opal ring on the spot. (She got a matching one when she had her first menstrual period.)

A few hours later, as I sat working at my typewriter, I heard my daughter yelling to me from the bathroom, "Hey, Mom, guess what I got twenty-one of?"

We had a pregnant cat at the time and, for a few horrible moments, I was struck numb with the thought of twenty-one kittens. But, it wasn't kittens. My daughter was back to counting pubic hairs.

The time that we'd spent learning about menstruation and puberty had paid off. My daughter had regained her sense of excitement about the changes that were taking place in her body. This healthy attitude toward her body alone made our discussions worthwhile, but there were also other changes. First of all, things between the two of us got much better. We were back to our old, easy footing. She didn't magically start cleaning her bedroom or anything like that. We still had our quarrels, but they subsided to a livable level. And when we fought, at least we were fighting about the things we said we were fighting about. The underlying resentment and tension that had been erupting from beneath even our mildest disagreements, engulfing us in volcanic arguments, was gone.

But the most amazing change, perhaps because it was so unexpected, was that my daughter's role in the playground machinations had begun to change. In *My Mother, My Self*, Friday suggests the mother's failure to deal with her daughter's dawning sexuality, her silence about menstruation and the changes in the daughter's body, is perceived by the daughter as a rejection of the daughter's feminine and sexual self.

This silent rejection of these essential elements of self, coming as it does just at the time in the daughter's life when these very aspects of femininity and sexuality are manifesting themselves in the physical changes of her body, is nothing short of devastating. The daughter feels an overwhelming sense of rejection from the figure in her life with whom she is most intensely identified. One of the ways in which the daughter seeks to cope, to gain some control over her emotional life, is through the psychodramas of rejection that she continually reenacts with her peers.

Or perhaps these dramas of rejection are more along the lines of the pecking-order behavior we see among chickens. The largest, boldest chicken pecks another smaller one away from the feed dish, that chicken retaliates by pecking on another smaller and more vulnerable chicken, and so on down the line. We cannot deal with mother's rejection directly by confronting her. We are too small, too vulnerable, too defenseless; so, in a classic case of displaced aggression, we turn around and attack another little girl. Or perhaps just the opportunity to act out rejection, whether we play the role of leader, follower, or victim, to make this devastating experience familiar, to carve out roles we at least know and are used to, provides some measure of relief.

Whatever the particular mechanism, I can't help but suspect that the cultural taboo about menstruation, a mother's ignorance of and reluctance to deal with the topic, and the phenomena of playground politics are inextricably tied up with one another.

One morning, sometime after my daughter and I had begun to return to our old footing, I was driving her to school when she started to talk about the problems she was having with her friends. I held my breath. This topic had become so volatile that I hadn't even broached it in months. I didn't want to say the wrong thing.

"I don't know what to do, Mommy," she told me. "I want to be Susan's and Tanya's friend, but they're always whispering and talking about Kathy, and they do it loud enough so she can hear. And I'm with them, but I really like Kathy too."

"Well, can't you be friends with everybody?" I said, biting my tongue almost as soon as I said it. This had been one of my stock replies whenever we had talked about the subject, and it usually caused a storm, but this time she merely answered me, "But if I don't get down on Kathy with them, Susan and Tanya won't be friends with me."

"So what do you do when that happens; how do you handle it?" I asked, trying to say something neutral.

"Well, I just kind of stand there. I don't actually say bad things about Kathy, but I'm there with Susan and Tanya, so it's like I'm against Kathy too. And it makes me feel terrible, like I'm not a very good person," she said, starting to cry. "I don't know what to do."

"Well, look," I said, "Susan and Tanya are both really nice girls. Why don't you just go up to them and say 'Look, I have a problem and it's really making me feel lousy,' and then just tell them what you told me—that you want to be their friend, but you don't dislike Kathy and it makes you feel lousy if you join in putting her down."

My daughter gave me a look that told me what she thought of my suggestion.

"Not such a good idea, huh?" I offered.

"No, Mom," she agreed, and I kissed her goodbye as the school bell rang. Maybe my advice wasn't much help. Maybe it wasn't even very good advice, but at least we'd talked about the subject with each other.

Two days later, when I picked her up from school, she told me, "Well, I tried doing what you said to do."

"How did it work?"

"It worked. Susan and Tanya said that it was okay, that they'd still be friends with me even if I didn't hate Kathy."

Big of them, I thought to myself, but I didn't say anything. In truth, I was pleased; my daughter had begun to carve out a new role in the game for herself.

Perhaps Nancy Friday was right. Maybe my daughter perceived my attention to the changes taking place in her body as an acceptance of her sexual self, and this, in turn, lessened her need to participate in these playground psychodramas of rejection. I didn't, and still don't, know whether Friday's theories are real explanations, but my experiences with my own daughter certainly seemed to validate her ideas. Still, I wouldn't want to go so far as to promise you that spending time teaching your daughter about menstruation and the other physical changes of puberty will magically deliver her from the psychodramatics of puberty or will automatically erase the tensions that so often exist between parents and their adolescent daughters. But my experiences with my own daughter and, more recently, as the teacher of a class on puberty and sexuality for teens and pre-teens, have convinced me that kids of this age need and want information about what is happening to them at this point in their lives.

This information isn't always easy to come by. Too often we parents simply don't have the facts to give our children. Most of us have, at best, a sketchy knowledge of menstruation, and it is a rare parent who can describe the five stages of breast or pubic hair development. This book was written to provide those facts.

The book is designed to be read by girls in the nine- to fifteen-year-old age group, but may also be appropriate for younger or older girls. It details the physiological changes in the female body during puberty. This book does not pretend to cover all the things you will need to discuss with your daughter as she goes through puberty. What book could? It is only a beginning.

ADDENDUM TO THE NEW EDITION

This book was first published in 1983. I revised and expanded the information four years later in response to the crucial issues raised by the AIDS epidemic, and the growing demand from parents and teachers for earlier and more extensive puberty and sex education for our youngsters.

The first eight chapters of this book, the ones that deal with the changes that are happening in children's bodies during puberty, are quite similar to those in the first edition. I have expanded the material on perspiration, pimples, shaving, and bras and made some other alterations here and there. But I haven't made any major revisions in these chapters. There simply wasn't any reason to do so, and I don't expect there ever will be. No matter how much the times may change, kids will undoubtedly continue to go through the same sequence of physical changes, and have the same questions, concerns, and anxieties about these changes generation after generation.

Thus, the major revisions in this new edition come later in the book. The original Chapter 9, which was a sort of catch-all chapter entitled "Sexuality," has been replaced with three new chapters: "Sexual Intercourse, Pregnancy and Childbirth, and Birth Control"; "Sexually Transmitted Diseases, AIDS, and Other Sexual Health Issues"; and "Romantic and Sexual Feelings." I decided to go into more detail on the subjects I'd only briefly mentioned in the original chapter for two reasons. First, I wasn't entirely satisfied with the original material; it was too sketchy. Indeed, in some cases, it seemed to raise more questions than it answered. Second, parents have encouraged me to go into greater detail about contraception, sexually transmitted diseases (in particular, AIDS), sexual decision-making, and other such topics. Some of these parents told me that they wanted to discuss these issues with their kids, but they weren't exactly certain what to say or how to say it. Similarly, others explained that they weren't sure *how much* to say or *when* (i.e., at what ages) to say it. Some said they'd looked for books that would discuss these subjects in more detail, but either they couldn't find one they liked, or the ones they liked were aimed at older teens. So parents, and teachers as well, urged me to write on these topics in a manner and style appropriate to my readership, that is, for kids in the nine- to fifteen-year-old age group.

Though I was flattered by such requests, I had some serious reservations about expanding the book in this way. I am disturbed by the tendency on the part of parents and educators to give kids *sex* education without first providing them with *puberty* education. It may sound like I'm splitting hairs here, but in my opinion puberty education and sex education are, or at least should be, distinct and separate things. There are, of course, areas of overlap between the two, but basically puberty education focuses on the physical and emotional changes that happen during puberty, while sex education focuses more on intercourse, contraception, the dangers of AIDS, rules for sexual conduct, and so forth.

In the wake of the teen pregnancy and AIDS epidemics, educators and parents are anxious to provide kids with more sex education and to start that education at younger ages than ever before. Schools all across the country have initiated "Just Say No" sex-ed programs (modeled after the drug abuse prevention programs) for seventh graders. The Surgeon General himself has recently suggested that AIDS education should begin as early as the third grade.

I suppose that, as someone who's been teaching in this underfunded, largely ignored, and even vilified field for the past ten years, I should be elated over this new enthusiasm and increased funding for sex education. But I'm not, for the fact of the matter is that less than two percent of seventh graders are sexually active, and the vast majority of third-graders are hardly at risk of developing AIDS. There is, no doubt, something to be said for beginning prevention programs early on. But I can't help feeling that much of this new push for more extensive and earlier sex education is more a reflection of adult anxieties about AIDS and adolescent sexual activity than it is a true concern with and understanding of the needs of children.

Elementary school children and seventh-graders don't need *sex* education, they need *puberty* education. Kids of this age have a multitude of questions and fears about the changes that are, or soon will be, taking place in their bodies. I get hundreds and hundreds of letters from kids, the envelopes covered with under-scored pleas—"Help!", "URGENT!", "Open At Once!", "Please! Please! Write Back Right Away!!!"—and inside there'll be five-page letters with intricate diagrams and lengthy explanations of some lump or bump or imagined physical abnormality that has the poor kid worried sick. These children need reassuring puberty education before they're ready for sex education.

When parents and schools ignore puberty education, which ad-dresses the true agendas of children, in favor of sex education, which is more apt to address the agendas of nervous adults, they are, in my opinion, missing the proverbial boat. Kids who aren't given reassuring puberty education when they need it do not re-spond as well to their parents' or schools' efforts to impart moral codes or even just safe, sane guidelines for sexual conduct.

I think it works something like this: Kids figure, "You were too embarrassed, too busy, too hung up on your own anxiety about my possible sexual activity to respond to my needs for information and reassurance about my changing body. Now, here you are, all freaked out about what I might be doing, trying to push your moral rules and sexual do's and don'ts at me. Well, you're too late. My sexuality is no longer any business of yours, I'm not going to listen to a word you say. So there."

When, on the other hand, kids are given puberty education, the dynamic is altogether different. It's been my experience that kids are enormously grateful for the reassurance they get from such education. I actually have had classes where kids burst into spon-taneous applause when I walked into the room. I also have a file drawer of touching letters from readers thanking me for having allayed some fear or doubt of theirs. Not only are kids grateful when their needs for reassurance are met in this way, but they also develop a profound respect for and trust in the source of that reassurance. Indeed, sometimes the wholesale nature of their trust is a bit unnerving, and I am not always entirely comfortable with the influence I seem to have, especially in situations that involve kids coming to me or writing to me for advice about whether they should become sexually active or how to handle an unplanned pregnancy.

But the point here is that parents need to realize they can forge a very powerful bond with their children if they will "be there" for them during puberty—not to mention how well the ensuing trust and respect will serve all concerned when it comes to later efforts at sex education.

You can see, then, why I had reservations about adding three chapters dealing largely with *sex* education issues to what is, first and foremost, a *puberty* education book. I was afraid that parents would tend to focus on the sex education aspects of the book and ignore the puberty education aspects, the first eight chapters.

Obviously, in the end, I did decide (for the reasons described earlier) to go ahead and add these new chapters. But unless your daughter is already through puberty, please don't let these new chapters become the sole, or even the main, focus of any conversations this book may generate between the two of you. Even if she herself tends to gravitate toward talking about the sexual issues, make the effort to steer your conversations back toward the physical and emotional changes of puberty.

Some tips on how best to go about talking with your daughter about puberty are probably in order here. First of all, be aware of the fact that you may have to initiate these conversations. As parents, we usually subject our kids to a constant stream of information and advice about virtually every aspect of their lives, from why they need to get a good education to what they should eat. But when it comes to anything having to do with sexuality, there's much less information and advice, perhaps even total silence. Our reticence or silence sends a message: It is not okay to talk about this topic. If this has been the case with you and your daughter, you'll have to put some effort into breaking this silence.

Second, remember that just one talk about puberty, or even a few, is not sufficient. Count the number of times in the last two weeks that you've discussed money, homework, irresponsibility, household chores, or another such topic with your daughter. Then count the number of times you've had a conversation about the physical or emotional changes of puberty and compare the scores. If you're batting zero, you need to work on improving your average.

Yet another piece of advice: Use a casual, spur-of-the-moment approach, rather than having formal, sit down, now-we're-going-to-discuss-puberty talks. Remember, too, that if any or all of these subjects is embarrassing for you, that's perfectly fine. Nowhere is it written: Thou shall not be embarrassed when discussing sexual topics with thine offspring. Most parents are embarrassed, especially when it comes to topics like masturbation. If you're embarrassed about any of these subjects, you can simply say something like, "Gee, this is so embarrassing for me, I can hardly talk about it. But I wished my parents had talked more to me and I don't want to let my embarrassment keep me from talking to you."

One more bit of wisdom: Avoid the direct, head-on approach. Saying things like "Do you have any questions about the things you've read in the book?" or "Would you like to talk about the changes happening in your body?" puts your daughter on the spot and probably won't work too well. Instead, take a slightly different tack. Pick an opportune moment and say something like, "When I was your age, I _____ ," and then fill in the blank with "started sprouting pubic hair and was worried because . . . ," "began developing breasts and felt . . . ," or with some misconception or embarrassing moment you had during adolescence. This is an almost sure-fire approach.

By virtue of your revelations about your own feelings or whatever dumb, embarrassing story you've told about yourself, you've let your daughter know: 1) that it is possible to survive puberty and even to eventually laugh about it; 2) that it's okay to be less-than-perfectly-all-knowing-and-confident about this whole business of puberty; and 3) that, lo and behold you, too, were young once— a fact that rarely impinges on most youngsters' minds. But, enough of these tips and back to the changes in this new edition.

Once I'd decided that I would, after all, add these new chapters, I found myself facing certain problems which I think are worth mentioning here. These stemmed from the fact that my readership covers such a wide age range—anywhere from age nine to fifteen or even older. This wasn't too much of a problem when the book dealt almost exclusively with puberty, but it presented difficulties in the new chapters.

Consider, for example, Chapter 11, which deals with romantic and sexual feelings. Older girls often have questions about dating or making decisions about sex, while younger girls may still be in the I-couldn't-care-less-about-boys stage. By the same token, issues such as how to handle the fact that your best friend is a boy are usually not very relevant to the lives of most fifteen-year-olds. So Chapter 11 had to cover a spectrum that began with questions about same-sex friendships and stretched all the way to questions about sexual decision-making. I realized that those whose questions fell on one end of the spectrum might not find the questions on the other end very interesting or applicable to their lives. I solved this problem by simply telling readers to skip any sections that didn't interest them, and I hope that you will also point this out to your daughter.

The wide age range was more problematic in the section on birth control in Chapter 9. The kind of contraceptive information that younger girls want or need is usually quite different from the sort of information that might be appropriate for a fifteen-year-old. Birth control isn't a major part of my curriculum for my younger classes, and the topic usually only comes up in response to questions in the class question box. Answering younger kids' questions is generally just a matter of correcting their mistaken ideas. (For example, they often think that taking birth control pills makes a woman infertile forever, and because they heard it called *The Pill*, they think it's about the size of a golf ball.)

Fifteen-year-olds, on the other hand, may have a much different level of interest and a much greater need for information. Twenty-two percent of the fifteen-year-old girls in this country are sexually active; thus, a girl of this age may well need specific, practical contraceptive advice. But she won't find it here.

Detailed, user-oriented birth control information would not only have been way over the heads of many of my readers, but including such information would have lengthened the book to the point where its sheer size alone would have scared off many younger or less able readers. So I made a compromise and, like most compromises, it isn't entirely satisfactory. The information here is appropriate for most of my readers. Still, there is probably more contraceptive information than a nine-year-old will want or need, and definitely less than a sexually active teen should have. So if you have an older daughter who is, or may be, sexually active, please don't rely on this book alone to meet her needs. At the very least, you should see that she gets (and reads) one of the books listed in the bibliography. If, on the other hand, you have a younger daughter (or for that matter a daughter of any age) who isn't interested in this topic or finds the information "over her head," she can, of course, skip it, although there's certainly no harm done if she were to go ahead and read it.

I know there are some parents who worry that giving kids access to information about birth control will encourage them to go out and experiment sexually. To such parents it seems patently obvious: The greater the availability of birth control, the greater the likelihood of kids having sex.

But adolescents' minds work differently, and to them, birth control and sexual activity are not necessarily linked. The average teenager is sexually active for at least a year before even considering using a method of birth control. Once they have a method, about two-thirds of them never use it or use it only sporadically. Besides, if birth control were causing teens to be sexually active, we wouldn't have upwards of a million teenage pregnancies each year, and we wouldn't be faced with the alarming statistic that four out of every ten of today's fourteen-year-olds will have been pregnant at least once by the end of their teen years. In the ten years that I've been working with kids, I have only known two (count 'em, *two*) girls who obtained a method of birth control *before* they started having sex. If you think teenagers are having sex because of the availability of contraception, you're putting the cart before the horse, at least by adolescents' logic. It just doesn't work that way.

So there is no harm done if your child should read the section on birth control, even though she may be way too young to have a practical need for it. Too many parents wait until their kids have begun dating or going steady to introduce the topic. Their first parent/child contraception conversations often come in the context of a parental message like, "I don't want you having sex yet, but if you do, I want you to use something." I think that's a perfectly legitimate message for a parent to send, but it's an awfully highly charged situation in which to initiate contraception education efforts, and kids are often confused by what sounds to them like a double message. It's much easier, less confusing to kids—and undoubtedly more effective—to begin discussions on birth control earlier.

Writing the section on sexually transmitted diseases in Chapter 10 posed problems similar to the ones I faced with birth control, and I made a similar sort of compromise. Younger readers may find more information than they need, and there may not be enough for sexually active readers. Here again, for the older girls, there are resources listed in the bibliography, and the younger readers can skip overly detailed material.

In my classes for older teens, I am quite frank and detailed, graphic even, in discussing AIDS and *all* the modes of transmission, for as the Surgeon General has so aptly put it, "You can't talk of the dangers of snake poisoning and not mention snakes." But in my classes for younger kids, I do not discuss the specific "high-risk" sex practice that, according to many experts, accounts for the high incidence of AIDS among male homosexuals. I'm not being coy in failing to say precisely which practice I am talking about here. I'm being deliberately obtuse because even younger kids sometimes read the parents' introductions to my books, and I don't think it's appropriate to discuss this high-risk practice with them. First of all, it's not necessary. In my experience, younger children's curiosity is quite satisfied with less specific explanations, and since they don't engage in this practice, there is no need to warn them against it. Second, all my instincts as a teacher tell me that a discussion of this high-risk sexual practice would be far too confusing and upsetting for many younger children.

At any rate, the AIDS discussion in this book is one that, to my mind, is appropriate for younger children. Those of you who feel the need for more explicit AIDS information will, I hope, make use of my new book for older teens, *Lynda Madaras Talks to Teens About AIDS.*

As in the first edition of this book, I have dealt with topics about which people have widely varying and often conflicting views. My approach to dealing with these topics is to present all the different opinions that people have, to explain why they have those views, and to do so in as fair and objective a manner as I can. I try very hard to honor the religious, moral, and ethical values of all parents, and I think I do a pretty good job of it. There may, however, be some parents who take exception to my approach. Some may object because they are so committed to their own values that they don't have any tolerance for anyone else's, and thus object to even the mention of alternate viewpoints on issues such as masturbation, abortion, or premarital sex. I'd venture to say that this simply isn't the right book for these parents. Other parents may object to my approach because they feel my personal values have colored what I've written, and they disagree with my opinions and values. There's undoubtedly some truth to this. But if you don't agree with something I've said, please don't, as the saying goes, "throw out the baby with the bathwater." Instead, take any objections you might have to what I've said as an opportunity to explain your own viewpoints and values to your child.

I hope this book will help you and your child develop an even closer and more loving relationship.

CHAPTER 1

Puberty

This book is about a time in a girl's life when her body is changing from a child's body into a woman's body. This time of changing is called *puberty*.

Our bodies change quite a bit as we go through puberty. We get taller. The general shape or contour of our bodies changes: Our hips and thighs get fleshier, and we take on a more rounded, curvy shape. Our breasts begin to swell and to blossom out from our chests. Soft nests of hair begin to grow under our arms

---

puberty (PEW-bur-tee)   The word *puberty* is pronounced with the accent on the first part of the word, PEW. You say that part of the word with the most emphasis. Throughout this book, there are a number of words that you may not have heard before. Whenever we use these words for the first time, we will include a pronunciation key like this at the bottom of the page.

and in the area between our legs. Our skin begins to make new oils that change the very feel and smell of us. At the same time that these changes are happening on the outside, other changes are taking place inside our bodies.

These changes don't happen overnight. Puberty happens slowly and gradually, over a period of many months or years. These changes may start when a girl is as young as eight, or they may not begin until she is sixteen or older. Regardless of when they start for you, you'll probably have a lot of questions about what is happening to your body. We hope that this book will answer at least some of these questions.

"We" are my daughter, Area, and I. The two of us worked together to make this book. We talked to doctors and research scientists and pored over medical textbooks. We also talked to mothers and daughters, to find out what happened to them during puberty, how they felt about it, and what kinds of questions they had. You'll hear their voices throughout this book. Some of the quotes in this book are from kids in my class. During the school year, I teach a class on puberty once a week at Sequoyah School in Pasadena, California. (My daughter used to go to Sequoyah, which is how I happen to be teaching there.) The kids in my class and the mothers and daughters we talked with had a lot of questions and a lot of things to say about puberty. So, in a sense, they too helped write the book.

I usually start the first puberty class of the year by talking about how babies are made. This seems like a good place to begin since the changes that occur during puberty happen to get the body ready for a time in our lives when we may decide to have a baby.

A talk with a group of boys and girls about how babies are made usually turns into a pretty giggly affair, because in order to talk about how babies are made, we have to talk about *sex*, and sex, as you may have noticed, is a *very big deal*. People often act embarrassed, secretive, giggly, or some other strange way when the topic of sex comes up.

Even the word itself is confusing, because *sex* can mean many different things and is used in different ways. In the simplest meaning of the word, *sex* refers to the different kinds of bodies that men and women have. There are a number of differences between male and female bodies, but the most obvious is that a male has a penis and scrotum and a female has a vulva and vagina. These body parts, or organs, are called *sex organs*. People are either members of the male sex or the female sex, depending on which type of sex organs they have.

The word *sex* is also used in other ways. We may say that two people are "having sex." Having sex, or *sexual intercourse*, involves a man putting his penis into a woman's vagina. Or we may say that two people are "being sexual with each other," which means that they are having sexual intercourse or that they are holding, touching, or caressing each other's sex organs. We may also say that we are "feeling sexual," which means that we are having feelings or thoughts about our sexual organs, about being sexual with another person, or about having intercourse.

Our sexual organs are very private parts of our bodies. We usually keep them covered up, and we don't talk about them in public very often. Having sex, being

penis (PEE-niss)
scrotum (SKRO-tum)
vulva (VUL-va)
vagina (vah-JIE-nah)
intercourse (IN-ter-korse)

sexual with someone, or having sexual feelings are also usually private matters that don't get talked about very often. So when I come into a classroom and start talking about penises and vaginas and having sex . . . well, things get pretty giggly. (You can imagine how my poor daughter felt, having her mother coming to school to talk about *those* things. Before I started teaching the class, I asked her if it was okay with her. She wasn't entirely happy with the idea. Finally she said all right, but no way was she going to be in the class! As it turned out, the classes were a big hit. Kids were coming up to her and saying how much they liked the class. So eventually she joined the class too, even though she'd heard most of this stuff at home.)

I decided that if we were going to get all silly and giggly in class when we talked about these things, we might as well get *really* silly and giggly. So, I start the first class of the year by giving everyone photocopies of the two drawings in Illustration 1 and red and blue colored pencils that we use to color the drawings.

Sex Organs

Illustration 1 shows the male and the female sex organs. These sex organs are also referred to as the *genitals,* or the *genital organs.* Everyone has sex organs on both the inside and the outside of the body, and they change as you go through puberty. These pictures show how the sex organs on the outside of the body look in grown men and women.

I generally begin with the male sex organs. I explain that the sex organs on the outside of a man's body have two main parts and that the scientific names for these parts are the *penis* and the *scrotum.* By the

genitals (JEN-a-tulls)

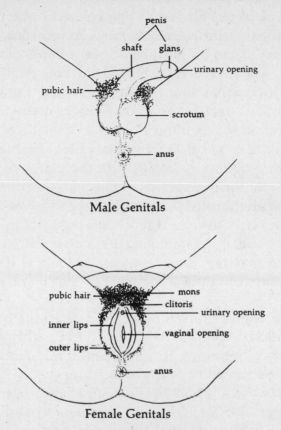

Male Genitals

Female Genitals

Illustration 1. The Genitals

time I've passed out the copies of the drawings and have started talking about the penis and the scrotum, the kids in my classes are usually giggling like mad, nudging each other, or falling off their chairs in embarrassment. I don't pay too much attention to how they're acting, I just say, "Okay, the penis itself also has two parts: the *shaft* and the *glans*. Find the shaft of the penis on your drawing and color it blue." Some kids keep giggling and some get more serious, but they all

glans (GLANZ)

start coloring. Why don't you color the shaft too (unless, of course, this book belongs to someone else or to a library. One of the people we admire most in the world is a wonderful lady named Lou Ann Sobieski. She's a librarian, and my daughter and I would be in very hot water if Lou Ann thought we were telling people to color on library books.)

After they've colored the shaft blue, I explain to my class that there is a small slit in the glans, right at the very tip of the penis, called the *urinary opening*. This is the opening through which urine (pee) leaves the body. I ask my class to color it red. Then we color in the glans itself. I usually recommend blue and red stripes, but color it any way you want, just as long as it's colored differently from the other parts so that it will stand out clearly.

Next comes the *scrotum*. "Red and blue polka dots for the scrotum," I tell my class. By this time, the picture is beginning to look rather silly, and the giggling has turned to outright laughter.

Inside the scrotum are two egg-shaped organs called *testes*, or *testicles*. You can't see them in these pictures, but I like to mention them at this point because they have a lot to do with making babies. We'll talk more about them in the following pages.

Then I ask the class to color in the pubic hair, the crisp, curly hairs that grow in the genital area. Finally, I ask my class to color the anus. The *anus* is the opening through which feces or bowel movements leave our bodies. It is not really a sex organ, but since it is located in the genital area, I like to mention it.

urine (YUR-in)
urinary (YUR-in-air-ee)
testes (TES-teez)
testicles (TES-ti-kuls)
pubic (PEW-bik)

The business of coloring in the different parts like this works well because it gets everyone laughing and makes it easier to deal with the nervousness many of us feel when we talk about sex organs. But I also have the kids do it for another reason: I think it helps them to learn the names of these organs. If you just look at the drawing and see that this part is labeled *penis* and that part *scrotum*, it's all kind of jumbled and doesn't stick in your mind. But if you spend a few moments coloring them in, you have to pay attention and you'll remember better. These are important parts of the body, so it's worth the effort. If this book isn't yours and you can't color in it, try making a tracing of these drawings and coloring on the tracings.

While everyone in the class is busy coloring pictures, we talk about slang words. People don't always use the scientific names for these body parts. The kids in my classes came up with quite a list of slang words for the penis, scrotum, and testicles.

SLANG WORDS FOR THE PENIS, SCROTUM, AND TESTICLES

PENIS		*SCROTUM AND TESTICLES*
cock	peter	balls
dick	rod	nuts
prick	dingus	eggs
schlong	dork	rocks
wee-wee	meat	jewels
wanger	pisser	cubes
pecker	hot dog	bags

Personally, I don't object to slang words, but some people do, and they may get upset if they hear you using them. You may or may not care about upsetting people in this way, but you should at least be aware of the fact that there are people who find slang words offensive.

When we've finished coloring the male sex organs, we move on to the female sex organs. The genital organs on the outside of a woman's body are sometimes referred to as the *vulva*. The vulva has many parts. We usually start at the top with the fleshy mound called the *mons*. Color it and the pubic hair blue. Then we move toward the bottom of the mons where it divides into two folds or flaps of skin called the *outer lips*. Try coloring them with red stripes. In between the outer lips lie the *inner lips*. Try blue stripes for the inner lips. The inner lips join together at the top, where there is a small, bud-shaped organ called the *clitoris*. Color it red. Just down from the clitoris, between the inner lips, is the urinary opening, the opening through which urine leaves the body. Color it blue. Below the urinary opening is another opening called the *vaginal opening*. It leads into the hollow pouch or cavity on the inside of our bodies called the *vagina*. Use your imagination—color the vaginal opening red, blue, polka dotted, striped, or whatever. Finally, we come to the anus; chose a color and color the anus.

While we're coloring in the female genitals, we also make a list of slang words used to refer to this part of a woman's body.

SLANG WORDS FOR THE VULVA AND VAGINA

cunt	muff	beaver	snatch
pussy	stuff	honeypot	poontang
	box	hole	

By the time we've finished coloring both these pictures, everyone has giggled off a good deal of their

mons (MONZ)
clitoris (KLIT-or-iss)
vaginal (VAH-jin-ul)

embarrassment. They have also gotten a pretty good idea of where these body parts are, which makes it a lot easier to understand how a man and a woman make babies.

Sexual Intercourse

When I tell the kids in my class what *sexual intercourse* means, they usually have two reactions. One is that they want to know just how a man's penis could get into a woman's vagina. I explain that sometimes the penis gets stiff and hard and stands out from the body. This is called an *erection*, and it can happen when a male is feeling sexual or is having sex with someone, and at other times too. (We'll say more about this later in the chapter "Puberty in Boys.") An erection happens because the spongy tissue inside the penis fills up with blood. Some people call an erection a "boner" or a "hard-on" because the penis feels so stiff and hard during an erection. It's almost as if there really is a bone in there. But there isn't any bone, just blood-filled, spongy tissue.

While it is erect, the penis can slide right into the vaginal opening. The vagina isn't very large, but it's very elastic and stretchy, so the erect penis can easily fit in there.

In addition to wanting to know *how*, some of the kids in my classes want to know *why* anyone would want to do this.

People have sexual intercourse for all sorts of reasons. It is a special way of being close with another person. It also feels good, which some of the kids in my class find hard to believe. But these areas of our

erection (e-REK-shun)

bodies have many nerve endings; if they are stroked or rubbed in the right ways, these nerve endings send messages to pleasure centers in our brains. When our pleasure centers are stimulated, we get pleasurable feelings all over our bodies. People also have sexual intercourse because they want to have a baby, but babies don't start to grow every time a man and woman have intercourse, just sometimes.

Making Babies

In order to make a baby, two things are needed: a seed from a woman's body, which is called an *ovum*, and a seed from a man's body, which is called a *sperm*.

Sperm are made inside the testicles, the two egg-shaped organs inside the scrotum. Sometimes, when a man and a woman are having sexual intercourse, the man *ejaculates*. When a man ejaculates, the muscles of the penis contract, and the sperm are pumped out of the testicles, through the *urethra* (the hollow tube in the center of the penis), and spurt out the opening in the center of the glans, as shown in Illustration 2. A teaspoonful or so of a creamy, white liquid, called *semen*, full of millions of tiny, microscopic sperm, comes out of the penis. This liquid is also called "ejaculate," or in slang terms "come" or "jism."

After the sperm leave the penis, they start swimming up toward the top of the vagina. They pass through a tiny opening at the top of the vagina that leads into an organ called the *uterus* (see Illustration 3). The uterus

ovum (OH-vum)
sperm (SPURM)
ejaculates (e-JACK-u-lates)
urethra (YUR-ree-thra)
semen (SEE-men)
uterus (YOU-ter-us)

is a hollow organ and, in a grown woman, it's only about the size of a clenched fist. But the thick, muscle walls of the uterus are quite elastic and, like a balloon, the uterus can expand to many times its size. The uterus has to be able to expand because it is here, inside a woman's uterus, that a baby grows.

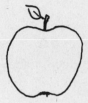

If you cut an apple in half, you would be able to see the seeds and core on the inside of the apple. This drawing, which shows the inside of an apple, is called a cross section.

The drawing below is also a cross section. It shows the inside of the penis and scrotum.

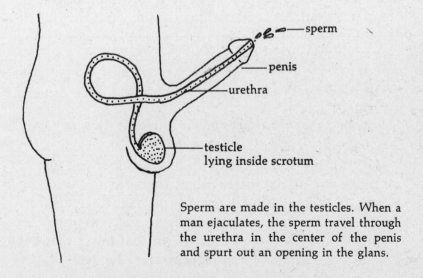

Sperm are made in the testicles. When a man ejaculates, the sperm travel through the urethra in the center of the penis and spurt out an opening in the glans.

Illustration 2. Cross Section of the Penis and Scrotum

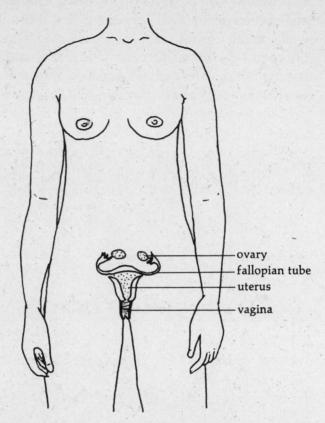

Illustration 3. The Sex Organs on the Inside of a Woman's Body

Some of the sperm swim up to the top of the uterus and into one of two little tubes, or tunnels, called the *fallopian tubes*. Not all the sperm make it this far. Some drift back down the uterus and out into the vagina where they join other sperm that never made it out of the vagina. These sperm and the rest of the creamy white liquid dribble back down the vagina and out of the woman's body.

fallopian (fuh-LOPE-e-an)

Women, too, make seeds in their bodies. When we are talking about just one of these seeds we use the word *ovum*. When we are talking about more than one, we use the word *ova*. The ova ripen inside two little organs called *ovaries*. In a young woman, the ovaries produce a ripe seed about once a month. When this seed is ripe, it leaves the ovary and travels down the fallopian tube toward the uterus. If a woman and man have sexual intercourse around the time of the month when the ripe ovum has just left the ovary, there's a good chance that the sperm and ovum will meet inside the tube. When a sperm and ovum meet, the sperm penetrates the outer shell of the ovum and moves inside it. This joining together of the ovum and the sperm is called *fertilization*, and when a sperm has penetrated an ovum, the ovum has been fertilized.

Most of the time, the ovum travels through the fallopian tube without meeting up with a sperm, and the tiny ovum just disintegrates. But, if the ovum has been fertilized, it doesn't disintegrate. Instead, the fertilized ovum plants itself on one of the inside walls of the uterus, and over the next nine months, it grows into a baby (see Illustration 4).

Menstruation

The inside walls of the uterus are covered by a special lining. Each month, as the ovum is ripening in the ovary, this lining gets ready just in case the ovum is going to be fertilized. The lining gets thicker. It also develops new blood passageways, for if the fertilized ovum plants itself in the lining, it will need plenty of rich

ova (OH-vah)
ovaries (OH-vah-reez)

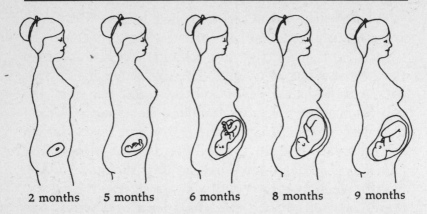

| 2 months | 5 months | 6 months | 8 months | 9 months |

Illustration 4. Stages of Pregnancy. A fertilized ovum plants itself on the inside wall of the uterus, and over the next nine months, it develops into a baby.

blood in order to grow and develop into a baby. Spongy tissues develop around these new blood passageways to cushion them. These tissues fill with blood and begin to make nourishment to help the ovum to grow.

If the ovum is not fertilized by meeting a sperm in the fallopian tube, then this newly grown lining in the uterus will not be needed. So, about a week after the unfertilized ovum has disintegrated, the uterus begins to shed this lining. The spongy, blood-filled tissue of the lining breaks down and falls off the wall. It collects in the bottom of the uterus and dribbles out into the vagina. It then flows down the length of the vagina and out the vaginal opening (see Illustration 5).

This breaking down and shedding of the lining inside the uterus is called *menstruation*. When the bloody lining dribbles out of the vaginal opening, a woman is menstruating or, as we say, having her period.

menstruation (mens-stroo-AY-shun)
menstruating (mens-stroo-AY-ting)

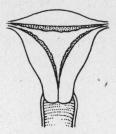

Each month, as the ovum is ripening in the ovary, the lining of the uterus gets thicker

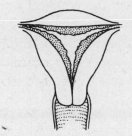

and thicker.

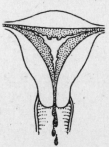

If the ovum is not fertilized, the lining begins to break down and dribble out of the body through the vagina.

Illustration 5. Cross Section of the Uterus. The shaded area is lining of the uterus.

The amount of blood that dribbles out during a period varies. Some of us have a couple of tablespoons, others have almost a cupful. The blood doesn't come out all at once, but dribbles out slowly over a number of days. Then it stops. It may only take a couple of days or it may take a week or so for all of the menstrual blood to empty out of your body.

Once the bleeding has stopped, the uterus starts growing a new lining in preparation for next month's ripe ovum. If that ovum is not fertilized, the newly grown lining will again break down, and you will have another period, usually within a month or so after your last period.

A girl may have her first period any time between her eighth and sixteenth birthdays. A few girls will have their first period when they are younger or older than this, but the majority of the girls have their first period between their eighth and sixteenth birthdays.

In the following chapters, we'll talk more about menstruation, about having your first period, and about the other changes that will take place in your body as you grow older and go through puberty. If you're like the kids in my class, you'll probably have a lot of questions about these things.

Everything You Ever Wanted to Know . . .

It isn't always easy to ask certain questions. We may feel too embarrassed to ask or we may feel our questions are just too dumb. If you've ever felt like this, you're not alone. In my classes, we play a game called "Everything You Ever Wanted to Know About Sex and Puberty, but Were Afraid to Ask." I pass out slips of paper at the start of each class so the kids can write down their questions and put them in a locked box. They don't have to sign their names to the questions, and I'm the only one who gets to see them, so nobody can look at the handwriting and figure out who wrote the question. I also leave the box in a place where people can get to it during the week in case they think up questions after class. At the end of each class, I take the questions out of the box, read them out loud, and answer them the best I can.

In writing this book, we've tried to answer all the questions that have come up in our "Everything You Ever Wanted to Know" game, but you may find that you have questions that aren't answered by this book. If so, perhaps your mom or dad, the school nurse, one of your teachers, or another adult can help you find answers to your questions. Or you could write to us. We'd love to hear about any questions or confusions you may have or about things you liked or didn't like about this book. Your envelope should be addressed like this:

Lynda Madaras
Newmarket Press
18 East 48th Street
New York, NY 10017

Be sure to include a self-addressed, stamped envelope so we can write back to you.

Using This Book

You may want to read this book with your parents, with a friend, or all by yourself. You may want to read it straight through from beginning to end, or you may want to jump around, reading a chapter here and there, depending on what you are most curious about. However you decide to go about reading this book, we hope that you'll enjoy it and that you'll learn as much from reading it as we did from writing it.

CHAPTER 2

Changing Size and Shape

If you notice that the jeans you bought just a couple of months ago are up around your ankles already or that your brand-new shoes are suddenly too small, it's probably because you are beginning to go through puberty. As you begin puberty, your body starts to grow at a faster rate.

The Growth Spurt

The sudden increase in the rate of growth at the start of puberty is called a "growth spurt." It happens at different ages for different girls, and is more noticeable in some girls than in others. It usually starts before you begin to develop breasts or to grow soft nests of hair in the area between your legs.

Starting around the age of two, the average girl grows about two inches a year until she starts puberty. When puberty begins, she may start growing twice as fast, so that she grows four inches that year instead of only two. Of course, not everyone is average, so you may grow more or less than this.

The growth spurt usually lasts less than a year, then the growth rate begins to slow down again. By the time you've had your first menstrual period, your growth rate has usually slowed back down to one or two inches a year. Most girls reach their full adult height within one to three years after their first period.

Boys go through a growth spurt during puberty too, but they usually don't start theirs until a couple of years after girls start. This is why eleven- and twelve-year-old girls are often taller than the boys their age. However, a couple of years later, when the boys start their growth spurt, they catch up to the girls and surpass them in height. Of course, some girls, the ones who are on the tall side, will always be taller than most of the boys. But often a girl who is taller than the boys she knows when she is eleven or twelve will find that the boys have caught up by the age of thirteen or fourteen.

During puberty, as you are growing taller, your bones are, of course, getting longer, but not all the bones in your body grow at the same rate. Your arms and legs tend to grow faster than your backbone during puberty, so you may notice that your arms and legs are longer in proportion to the trunk of your body than they were during childhood or than they will be when you reach adulthood.

The bones in your feet also grow faster than your other bones. Thus, your feet reach their adult size long before you've reached your adult height. A number of the girls we talked to worried about this. As one girl explained:

> I was just a little over five feet tall when I was eleven, but I wore a size eight shoe. I thought, Oh, no, if my feet keep on growing, they're gonna be gigantic! But I'm sixteen now, and I'm five feet eight inches tall, but my feet are still size eight.

In reaction to this, another girl said:

> I'm sure glad to hear that. I wear a size eight and a half now and I'm only twelve years old and five foot one and a half. People are always teasing me about my big feet. The last time I got tennis shoes, the guy in the store made some big joke about how if my feet got any bigger, he'd have to sell me the shoe boxes to wear. I pretended to laugh, but I was embarrassed and worried that maybe my feet were just going to keep getting bigger and bigger.

Changing Contours

As you go through puberty, your face changes. The lower part of your face lengthens and your face gets fuller. The general shape or contour of your body also changes. Your hips get wider as fat tissue grows around the hips, buttocks, and thighs so your body begins to have a rounder, curvier shape (see Illustration 6). Your breasts are also developing fat tissue, so they too get rounder and fuller. (We'll talk more about breasts in Chapter 4.)

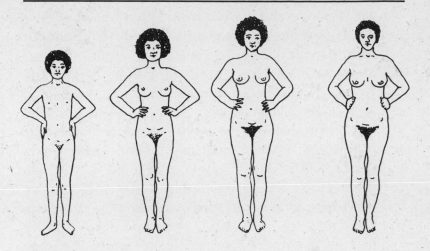

Illustration 6. Girls in Puberty. As we go through puberty, our hips get wider. Fat tissue begins to grow around our hips, thighs, and buttocks, giving our bodies a curvier shape. Our breasts begin to swell, and soft nests of hair begin to grow under our arms and around our genitals.

Liking Your Own Shape

Bodies come in all sorts of shapes and sizes—short or tall, thin or plump, narrow or wide, angular or curvy, straight or rounded. To some extent, you can change the shape of your body by diet and exercise. If you are thin, you can put on weight. If you are fat, you can diet so that your body loses some of its fat tissue. You can exercise to build up or slim down areas of your body. But you do have a basic shape to your body that can't be changed, no matter how much or how little you eat or what kind of exercise you do.

If you aren't satisfied with your body and are under- or overweight, perhaps you need to see a doctor and get on a diet and exercise plan to help you gain or lose weight. If you are not sure whether you're under- or overweight, your doctor can help you decide if your weight is within normal ranges for your height and body build. If you fall within these weight ranges and still aren't happy with the way your body looks, maybe you need to think about where you've gotten these ideas about how your body *should* look that are making you feel dissatisfied with the way you do look.

It would be nice if we could all just look at our bodies without having to compare them to someone else's and just say, "Hey, I like the way I look." But we live in a society where there's a lot of competition between people, between companies, and even between countries. We are always comparing and competing to see who's best. But who decides what's best?

Most of us get our ideas about what's the "best" or "most attractive" kind of female body from the pictures we see in magazines and billboards and from television and movies. Right now, in our country, these pictures usually show tall, thin, blond, blue-eyed, white-skinned women with rosy cheeks, no pimples or freckles, flat stomachs, tiny waists, long legs, big breasts, hairless legs and underarms, curvy hips and thighs—without a single bulge anywhere. As you may have noticed, there are few of us who actually look like this. For one thing, we aren't all white-skinned, blond-haired, and blue-eyed. And we aren't all thin with tiny waists and big breasts. We come in a pleasing array of sizes, shapes, and colors.

But when we are constantly bombarded with pictures of these glamorous images of slender, blond, blue-eyed women, it can make us feel that there is something about our hips, breasts, thighs, height, shapes, faces, skin, or hair that is somehow not right.

If we don't look like these women, we may be unhappy with the way we look. In fact, people in this country are often so unhappy about their looks that they spend millions and millions of dollars each year on hair dyes, makeup, fad diets, leg and underarm hair removers, tummy flatteners, breast developers, waist trimmers, and on and on. Some people even have operations to make their tummies flatter, their noses straighter, or their breasts a different size.

With all the images of these "perfect" women who seem to be having glamorous lives and no problems at all, it's easy to get to thinking that these kinds of bodies actually *are* better or more attractive. If you get to feeling that way sometimes, it might help you to remember these bodies only seem to be more desirable because they are in fashion in our particular culture at this particular time. Being in fashion doesn't make a mini-skirt "better" than a knee-length skirt, and being in fashion doesn't make one body type "better" than another.

It helps, too, to remember that fashions change and that they vary from culture to culture. The drawings you see in Illustration 7 show bodies that have been in fashion in other times and in other cultures. The first drawing is a flapper from America in the 1920s. During the 1920s in this country, curvy bodies and big breasts were definitely not in fashion. In fact, women with big breasts wrapped their breasts tightly, strapping them down, so that they wouldn't stick out. The second drawing shows a woman from Europe in the 1500s. Today she would be considered a bit chunky, but back then her type of body was the "best," "most attractive" kind of body a woman could have. The third drawing shows a Polynesian woman. She hardly matches our culture's standard of beauty, but in her culture, she'd

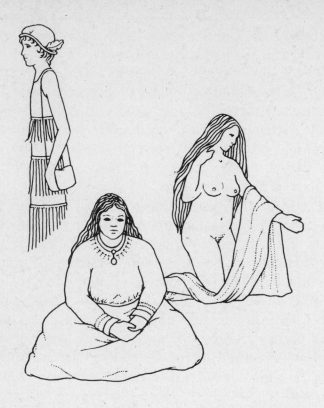

Illustration 7. Types of Beauty. From the top, clockwise, are a flapper, a woman from the 1500s, and a Polynesian woman.

be considered a great beauty and her rounded body would be considered the "best" and "most attractive."

Learning to appreciate yourself and to love your own body, regardless of whether or not it matches up with what's in fashion, is a big step in growing up. And if you can manage to find your own body attractive, other people will too, and it won't matter whether it's the so-called best or most attractive kind of body— not one bit. We guarantee it.

CHAPTER 3

Body Hair, Perspiration, and Pimples

For some girls, the growth spurt and the changes in the shape of their bodies are the first signs of puberty. For others, the first sign that puberty is beginning is that they start growing hair in new places on their bodies.

Pubic Hair

Pubic hair is the name given to the curly hairs that grow in the area of our bodies where our legs join together. This area has many names, such as the vulva or the genital area. Some people call this area of the body the vagina. Actually, the vagina is inside your body, so it is not really correct to call it the vagina.

pubic (PEW-bik)

If you stand sideways in front of a mirror, you'll notice that there is a little mound of flesh in this area that protrudes (sticks out) a bit. This mound is called the *mons*, which is a word from Latin that means little hill or mound. It is also called the *mons veneris*. *Veneris* is another Latin word that refers to Venus, the goddess of love, so *mons veneris* means "mound of Venus" or "mound of love." The mons is just one part of the vulva or genital area. We'll be talking about the other parts of the vulva later, but for now, let's concentrate on the mons.

The mons is a pad of fat tissue that lies under the skin. It cushions the pubic bone that lies beneath it. If you press down on the mons, you can feel the pubic bone underneath. For this reason, the mons is also referred to as the *pubis*. Regardless of what you call it, sooner or later you will begin to notice curly, colored hairs growing here.

If you look at your mons, you will notice that, toward the bottom, it divides into two folds or flaps of skin. These are the *labia majora*, or outer lips. In many girls, pubic hair first begins to grow on the edges of these lips. In others, it first begins growing on the mons itself.

Five Stages of Pubic Hair Growth

Doctors have divided pubic hair growth into the five different stages shown in Illustration 8. You may be in one of these stages or in between one stage and another. See if you can find the stage you're closest to.

veneris (ven-AIR-iss)
pubis (PEW-bis)
labia (LAY-bee-uh)
majora (may-JOR-ah)

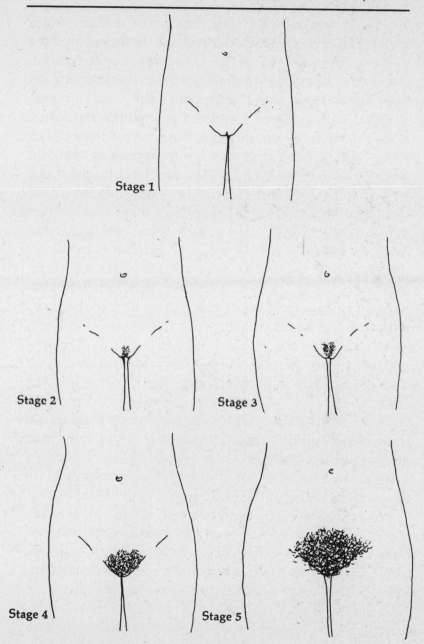

Illustration 8. The Five Stages of Pubic Hair Growth

Stage 1 starts when you are born and continues throughout childhood. In this stage the mons and the lips are either hairless or they have a few light-colored, soft hairs similar to the hair that may be growing on your belly. There aren't any pubic hairs.

Stage 2 starts when you grow your first pubic hairs. If you have hairs growing on your vulva during childhood, you will be able to tell the difference between these childhood hairs and pubic hairs because the pubic hairs are longer, darker in color, and curly. At first, they may be only slightly curly and there may be just a few of them. You may have to look very closely in order to see them.

In Stage 3, the pubic hairs get curlier and thicker, and there are more of them. They may get darker in color. They cover more of the mons and the lips than they did in Stage 2.

In Stage 4, the pubic hair gets still thicker and curlier, and it may continue to get darker in color. It also spreads out so it covers more of the mons and the lips.

Stage 5 is the adult stage. The pubic hair is thick and coarse and tightly curled. It covers a wider area than in Stage 4. It usually grows in an upside-down triangle pattern. In some women, the pubic hair grows up toward the belly button and out onto the thighs.

You may start growing pubic hair when you are only eight, or you may not start until you are sixteen or older. Most girls get to Stage 3 between the ages of eleven and thirteen. Most girls have their first menstrual period when they are in Stage 4, but many start their periods while they are still in Stage 3. A few will start their periods while they are only in Stage 2, and a few others won't start until after they've reached Stage 5. If you start your period while you are still in Stage 1 and your breasts haven't started to develop either, then you should see a doctor. Starting your period before you have any pubic hair and before your breasts have begun to develop doesn't necessarily mean that something is wrong, but it may mean that you have a problem. So you should see a doctor and get it checked out.

Color and Amount of Pubic Hair

Some women have lots of pubic hair, while on others, it is sparse. It may be blond, brown, black, or red and does not necessarily match the color of the hair on your head. The hair on your head may turn gray when you get old, and your pubic hair may also turn gray.

Why Pubic Hair?

One of the questions the girls in my class often ask is why we have pubic hair. Pubic hair helps keep the area between our labia majora, or outer lips, clean. Just as our eyelashes catch dust, dirt particles, or other things that could irritate our eyes, so our pubic hair catches things that could irritate the sensitive area between our outer lips. During childhood, we don't need the protection the pubic hair provides because this area is not as sensitive as it becomes during puberty.

Feelings About Pubic Hair

Some of the girls we talked to felt really excited about growing pubic hairs. Here's what one girl had to say:

> One day I was taking a bath and I noticed three little curly hairs growing down there. I started yelling for my mom to come and see. I felt real grown up.

Other girls weren't sure what was happening. As one girl explained.

> I saw these curly, black hairs and I didn't know what they were, so I got the tweezers and pulled them out. Pretty soon, they grew back, and then there were more and more of them. So I figured it must be okay.

Growing pubic hair can be pretty scary, especially if you don't know what's happening. A number of girls told us that they plucked their first pubic hairs. It's not really a very good idea to pluck your pubic hairs. For one thing, they'll just grow back. Also, plucking them could cause the skin to get irritated, sore, or infected (not to mention the fact that plucking them could be very painful).

Although many of the girls we talked to felt excited about beginning puberty, not all of them were. Some of the girls didn't like the fact that they were growing pubic hair and going through the other changes of puberty. One girl had this to say:

> I just wasn't ready. I remember when I first saw that my pubic hairs were growing. I thought, Oh, no, I don't want this to start happening to me yet. Then I got breasts and it was like I suddenly started having this grown-up body, but I still felt like a kid inside.

Another girl said that she was excited and proud about her body maturing, but at the same time, she was also uncertain:

> I was afraid I was going to have to be all grown up and wear high heels all the time instead of being a tomboy and climbing trees. But, really, it turned out that I did just the same things I always did.

All the girls we talked to, whether they felt good or bad (or a bit of both) about the changes happening in their bodies, agreed that it helps to have someone to talk to about your feelings. Reading this book with someone might be a good way of starting to talk about those things.

Underarm Hair

We also start to grow hair under our arms during puberty. Most girls don't start growing underarm hair until after they've started growing pubic hair or their breasts have started developing. Many don't grow underarm hair until after their first period. But for a few girls, underarm hair is the very first sign that puberty is beginning. Although this is unusual, it's not abnormal, and it doesn't mean there's anything wrong. The other changes, developing pubic hair and breasts and having your first period, will all happen eventually.

Other Body Hair

The hair on our arms and legs may get darker as we go through puberty, and we may have more of it than we did during childhood. Some girls notice that they begin to grow darker hairs on their upper lips as well.

Shaving

In some parts of the world, women with lots of underarm and leg hair are considered more attractive or more womanly than women who don't have much hair on these parts of their bodies. In our country, the opposite seems to be true, at least in many people's minds. Here it seems that women who don't have hair on their underarms or legs are considered more attractive. The pretty, glamorous women we see in magazines, on TV, and in the movies have smooth, hairless legs and armpits. It's not that these women are somehow different from us and don't grow hair in these places. They are hairless because they shave their hair or they remove it by using chemical hair removers or by some other means.

Boys start growing hair under their arms and on their legs during puberty too. When boys start growing hair in these places, they generally feel very proud. It is a sign that they are turning from boys into men. On men, leg and underarm hair is considered attractive and manly. On women, it is often considered unattractive and unfeminine, which doesn't make much sense if you think about it.

You'll have to decide for yourself whether or not you want to remove the hair from your legs and underarms. It's not always easy to make this decision on your own because of pressure from the people around you, as in this girl's case.

> I wasn't going to shave my legs, but then my girlfriends started saying, "Oh, gross, look at all the hair on your legs. How come you don't shave it?" So I started doing it even though I didn't really want to.

Some girls said that they wanted to shave their legs, but their mothers said they couldn't. If your mom doesn't want you to shave and you want to, that's something you and she will have to work out between you. Your decision should be your own, though, without pressure one way or another from someone else. (We hope this last statement doesn't get us in trouble with too many moms.)

If you do decide to remove hair from your legs, armpits, or upper lip, there is something you should know before you start: once you start removing hair, it tends to grow back darker and thicker. So, after awhile some women find that they have to remove it every couple of days if they want to stay smooth and hairless.

There are basically four ways of removing hair: by shaving with a razor, by using a chemical cream remover (a depilatory), by using a wax remover, or by electrolysis.

You can use a razor to remove hair from your legs or underarms. But don't use a razor to remove hair from your upper lip, as this may eventually leave a stubble or a darkened area on your lip. You can use an electric razor or a regular one to shave your legs or armpits. Make sure the blades are smooth and free of nicks, or you may cut yourself. A dull blade can pull, or "drag," on your skin, so make sure you use a sharp one. It's pretty hard to cut yourself with an electric razor, but it's not at all hard to cut yourself with a regular one, so go easy. Use soap or shaving cream and always shave in the direction of hair growth to reduce the drag of the razor on your skin.

Chemical cream hair removers kill the hair at the root. You put the cream on and leave it there for a certain amount of time. When you wipe it off, the hair comes off, too. Don't use them on your armpits as you could get badly irritated or infected armpits. Certain types of chemical removers can be used on your upper lip, but *never* use a chemical hair remover that is intended for your legs on your face. It could badly irritate the facial skin. Also, be sure to follow the directions and

electrolysis (e-LEK-TROL-eh-sis)
depilatory (de-PILL-eh-tor-ee)

test the cream for an allergic reaction on a small area of skin before using it.

Another way of removing hair is to heat wax and spread it on the area where you want the hair removed. When the wax is cool, you pull it off and the hairs pull off along with the wax. Wax kits are available at your local drugstore. Some are designed for use on the legs, some on the face, and some on the bikini line (see below). Still other kits are made to be used in all these areas. Read the instructions carefully and be sure you use the wax *only* on the area for which it is intended.

Electrolysis is a more permanent method of removing hair, although in most cases the hair does eventually grow back. Electrolysis involves the use of an electric current to destroy the hair root. It is generally used for removing facial hair. Electrolysis should only be done by someone trained in the technique. Your doctor may be able to help you find someone trained in electrolysis.

Since high-cut bathing suits and bikinis have become fashionable, many girls have asked us about the best way to remove pubic hair so that it won't show under these new-style swim garments. As we explained earlier, plucking pubic hair *is not* a good idea. Nor is it a good idea to use a chemical cream remover on this area of your body. You can shave your "bikini line" with a razor, but go easy, use plenty of shaving cream, and always shave down, in the direction of hair growth. Even if you do this you may find that shaving still leaves unsightly red bumps and irritated skin. So, if you want to shave your bikini line, experiment by shaving a small area, and then waits at least twenty-four hours to make sure you don't have a bad reaction. There are also wax removers—"bikini wax kits"—that can be used in this area of the body. However, make sure that the wax you use is intended for use in this area of your body and always follow the directions carefully.

Perspiration and Body Odor

Another change you may notice as you go through puberty is that you begin to have more perspiration (sweat) under your arms. This happens because your sweat glands become more active during puberty. The odor of your underarm perspiration may also change, so that you have a more adult odor. You may also notice that other areas of your body—such as your feet, or your vulva—have more perspiration and a different odor. Or, you may notice that the palms of your hands, which contain numerous sweat glands, tend to perspire more or to get rather clammy from time to time.

Although these changes in perspiration and body odor are natural and healthy and are another sign that you are growing up, some young people worry about the odor and the increase in perspiration. Actually, it's not so surprising that some young people worry about these things. Advertising agencies spend millions of dollars each year on TV commercials and magazine ads designed to make us worry about our body odors and whether or not we're "dry" enough. But if you're healthy and eat properly, your body odor shouldn't be offensive. Bathing or showering regularly and wearing freshly laundered clothing should keep you smelling clean and fresh. If you perspire quite a bit and this bothers you, you may find that wearing 100 percent cotton underwear will help. Cotton is more absorbent than synthetic (man-made) materials. Wearing outer shirts and pants or skirts made of cotton or wool or other natural fibers also may help.

We all tend to perspire more when we're nervous. During puberty, this tendency may be even more noticeable. Lots of teenagers get clammy hands or break out in a sweat when they become nervous. This is perfectly normal and usually lessens after you reach your twenties. Sometimes just admitting to yourself, "Yes, I'm feeling really nervous (or embarrassed or uptight) right now," will help you relax and perspire less.

Deodorants and Antiperspirants

If you are bothered by the odor or amount of your underarm perspiration, you may want to use a deodorant or an antiperspirant. There are a number of these products on the market. They come in aerosol cans, non-aerosol sprays, sticks, creams, roll-ons—you name it. Some are "unscented," and some have a scent added to cover up the smell of the product. Some are advertised as being especially for men (or women), but generally there isn't much difference between a so-called man's deodorant and a woman's deodorant.

Underarm deodorants are aimed at covering up your body odor with the supposedly more pleasant odor of the deodorant. Antiperspirants also contain a substance to dry up perspiration. The most effective antiperspirants contain aluminum chlorohydrate. Some people think that the aluminum can soak through your skin and get into your bloodstream, and that this may be harmful. Other people disagree. You'll have to decide for yourself whether you want to use this kind of product.

Whatever you decide, be sure to read the label. Some products work best when you use them at bedtime rather than first thing in the morning. You may find that it is better not to put on deodorant or antiperspirant just after you jump out of a hot bath or shower. If you perspire afterwards, the deodorant or antiperspirant may just wash away. It might be better to let your body cool down a bit first.

While we're on the subject of body odor and deodorants, we want to say something about your vulva and about vaginal deodorant sprays. You have sweat glands in your vulva and these, too, become more active during puberty. In addition, you have oil glands in your vulva, which also become more active. The increase of activity of these oil and sweat glands may make your vulvar area feel more moist and have a different odor than when you were younger. Nowadays there are vaginal deodorant sprays made for use on your vulva, however, we don't recommend them because they can irritate the vulva. Besides, unless you have an infection, your vulvar area shouldn't have an unpleasant smell. Daily washing with soap and water and clean cotton underwear is all it takes to keep you smelling fresh. If you have a strong-smelling discharge from your vagina, or if your vulva smells badly, you may have an infection, and you should see a doctor rather than covering up the odor with a vaginal deodorant. (For more information on vaginal infections, see Chapter 10 on sexually transmitted diseases).

Pimples, Acne and Other Skin Changes

The oil glands in your skin also become more active during puberty. Your skin becomes more oily, and for many young people, this leads to skin problems like pimples and acne. Some kids have only mild problems

acne (AK-nee)

with their skin; others have more severe problems; still others don't have any problems at all. But eight out of every ten teenagers have at least mild skin problems.

Pimples and other skin disturbances happen during puberty because your oil glands begin to make excess amounts of an oily substance called *sebum*. You have oil glands throughout your skin, all over your body. They are especially numerous on your face, neck, shoulders, upper chest and back. Sebum is made in the lower part of an oil gland and travels through the duct (or neck) of the gland to a pore, a tiny opening on the surface of your skin. Sebum helps keep our skin soft and pliable.

However, if you produce too much sebum, the pore may become clogged, and a blackhead may form. A lot of people think that blackheads are little particles of dirt trapped in the pores. This isn't true. Blackheads are black not from dirt, but because the sebum and other substances produced by the glands sometimes turn black when they come in contact with the oxygen in the air.

Some young people get whiteheads, which are also the result of sebum. The sebum gets trapped just below the surface of the skin and forms the small, raised, whitish bumps we call whiteheads.

If blackheads are not removed, the sebum may continue to fill the duct. This may cause pressure, irritation, and inflammation. Germs can get in the duct and cause an infection. Whiteheads can also become inflamed and infected. Pimples—red bumps that may be filled with whitish pus—can develop. If you have a serious case of infected pimples, you have a problem called *acne*. Acne can be very troublesome and may cause pitting or scarring of the skin.

sebum (SEE-bum)

Pimples and acne are often more of a problem for those who naturally tend to have a more oily type of skin. The oiliness of your skin type, plus the increased oil you produce during puberty, combine to make you a candidate for these kinds of skin problems. If you have oily skin and pimples or acne during your teenage years, you may find yourself wishing you had drier, less acne-prone skin. But when you're older, you may be glad to have oily skin, because this type of skin doesn't wrinkle as easily as dry skin does.

Acne also tends to "run in families," so if your parents or older brothers and sisters had acne, you may be more likely to develop it. Many doctors believe that eating certain foods—chocolate, salty foods like nuts and chips, greasy foods—make a person more susceptible to acne. However, other doctors disagree. In one study, the amount of chocolate eaten didn't seem to have anything to do with acne. Still, if you find that certain foods give you pimples, it's best to avoid those foods.

Stress may also be a factor in acne. Many teenagers find that they "break out" (that is, get a lot of pimples) just before an important event—a dance, a big date, a match—that they're particularly nervous or excited about.

Although sunlight may have a beneficial effect on pimples and acne and many help to "dry out" your skin, it can also aggravate the problem. In a hot, dry climate, the sunshine may be helpful. However, hot, humid climates may make pimples and acne even worse. Some teenagers sit under a sunlamp to help dry out their acne and/or to get a tan. This isn't always a good idea. For one thing, sitting under a sunlamp can cause a severe sunburn, even if you stay there only for a minute more than the recommended time. While you're under the lamp, it may not seem like much is happening, so it's tempting to stay longer. All too often, this results in red, sunburned skin the next day. If you do use a sunlamp, *follow the instructions carefully*.

Another problem with sunlamps or, for that matter, with prolonged sunbathing, is that it can cause your skin to age before its time. People who have spent a lot of time in the sun or under sunlamps often develop wrinkles sooner, making them look older than they are. Overexposure to sunlight also increases your chances of getting skin cancer later in life. So be sure to go easy on the sun and tanning treatments.

Acne and pimples are most common between the ages of fourteen and seventeen, although they also happen to older and younger boys and girls. Some teenagers are troubled by acne for only a year or two. Then their oil glands adjust, their skin becomes less oily, and their acne and pimples clear up. Others have these problems throughout their teenage years. For a few young people, acne continues to be a problem even after their teens.

Kids often want to know if there is anything they can do to prevent pimples or to cure acne. Although there aren't any foolproof ways to prevent pimples, or any 100 percent effective cures for acne, there are some things that help. Frequent shampoos will keep greasy, oily hair from adding to the oil on your skin. Washing the especially oily areas—your face, neck, shoulders, back, and upper chest—at least once a day may also help prevent pimples. Washing removes the oil from the surface of the skin and helps keep your pores open. Wash with warm water, which helps open your pores, and rinse with cool water to close the pores up again. Wiping with a cotton ball or pad soaked in an alcohol-based astringent after you wash will remove any leftover oil and dirt. (You can buy isopropyl alcohol for under a dollar a bottle at drugstores.) You can also buy special presoaked pads, but they're usually rather expensive. Go easy on the alcohol, though. It can remove too much oil and leave your skin very dry.

·If you have especially oily skin, you may want to wash two or three times a day with ordinary soap. One of the antibacterial soaps sold in drugstores may also be helpful. (Ask the druggist to recommend one.) If you have pimples on your back, shower once or twice a day using an antibacterial soap and a back brush to scrub.

If you have blackheads, an abrasive soap or cleanser may help. (Again, ask your druggist to recommend one.) The abrasive in the soap often opens your pores and removes the blackheads. Be careful, though, because these soaps can irritate your skin. Don't use them more often than the instructions recommend. Also, black teenagers should avoid abrasives because their skin has a tendency to develop lighter or darker patches in the areas on which they've used the abrasives.

Washing, even with antibacterial soaps or abrasives, isn't always enough to prevent pimples and acne. Occasionally, mild cases of acne can be cleared up by using medicated acne lotions and creams that are sold without prescription. If these medications and the washing routines we've described don't take care of your problem and you're really bothered by acne, ask your doctor to refer you to a *dermatologist*, a doctor who specializes in skin problems.

Very often, parents say, "Oh, your skin doesn't look that bad," or "Leave it alone, you'll outgrow it." But if you take the time to explain to your parents how

isopropyl (ICE-eh-PRO-pill)
dermatologist (DUR-meh-TOL-e-jist)

much your skin problems bother you, they'll probably listen.

What can a dermatologist do for you? Well, that depends. If blackheads are a problem, the doctor can use a device called a comedo extractor to remove the blackheads (*comedo* is the scientific term for blackhead). The comedo extractor exerts pressure on the skin and causes the blackhead to pop out of the pore, thus unclogging the duct. The area around the blackhead may be a little red for a while, but unlike squeezing or "popping" your blackheads with your fingers, the comedo extractor won't leave scars. You should never pop your blackheads or pimples because you might end up with permanent scars or pits. The extractor is used only on blackheads. Once you've got an actual pimple, using the extractor may cause more harm than good.

The dermatologist can also prescribe drugs that are more effective than the medications you can buy without a doctor's prescription. For example, in certain cases, the dermatologist may prescribe a drug called *tetracycline*. Tetracycline is an antibiotic that kills germs and can fight the infections that often start in clogged pores and lead to acne. This drug also cuts down on the amount of sebum your oil glands produce. For some teenagers tetracycline works miracles and completely cures their acne. However, you should only use it under a doctor's supervision because in some people it can cause problems, such as upset stomach and increased sensitivity to sunlight (sunburns). These and other side effects are usually pretty mild but you must follow your doctor's orders carefully. There are also other treatments a doctor can prescribe, so if you are

comedo (KOM-eh-DOE)
tetracycline (TET-reh-SIGH-clean)

seriously troubled by skin problems, do see a dermatologist.

Stretch Marks

Some young people develop stretch marks, purplish or white lines on their skin, during puberty. This isn't common, but it does happen. It happens because the skin is stretched too much during rapid growth, and it loses its elasticity, or stretchiness. (Other things, such as taking certain medications, being pregnant, or gaining a lot of weight, can also cause stretch marks.) Many times these marks will fade or get less noticeable as a person gets older.

Pubic hair, underarm hair, perspiration, and skin changes are just a few of the changes you may notice in your body as you go through puberty. In the next chapter, we'll be talking about yet another change— the change in your breasts.

CHAPTER 4

Boobs, Boobies, Knockers, Melons, Jugs, Tits, and Titties: Your Breasts

Eskimos have over a hundred words for snow in their language because snow is such an important part of their lives. Judging from the number of words we have for breasts—the boys and girls in my class came up with dozens—breasts must be an important part of our lives.

I no longer remember exactly when I first noticed that my breasts were beginning to develop, but I sure remember the first time someone else noticed. I was baby-sitting for some friends of my parents who had nine-year-old twin girls. It was the first time I'd ever baby-sat for these girls. (It was also the last time. They dumped their pet guppies in the toilet, "so the guppies would have more room to swim around." While I was on my hands and knees fishing the guppies out of the toilet bowl, they were down in the kitchen putting their miniature turtle into the toaster, "to get it warmed up.")

The evening got off to a bad start. They were nice as pie while their mom and dad were there, but as soon as the door closed behind their parents, they jumped on me, pulling open my blouse: "Oh, you've got titties. Let's see, let's see," they demanded. "We can't wait till we get titties."

I managed to get the two of them off me and to button up my blouse, but I had never been so embarrassed in my life.

Regardless of whether you're as eager as those two twins or as mortified as I was, sooner or later your breasts will begin to develop.

The Breast During Childhood

When we are children, our breasts are flat, except for a small, raised portion in the center of each breast called the *nipple*. The nipple can range in color from a light pink to a brownish black and is surrounded by a

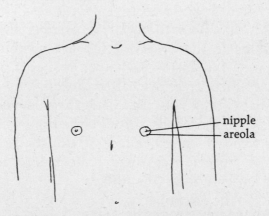

Illustration 9. The Breast. In the center of each breast is a small raised part called the "nipple," which is surrounded by a ring of skin called the "areola."

nipple (NIP-pull)

ring of flesh of about the same color that is called the *areola* (see Illustration 10).

Sometimes, when our breasts are touched or stroked or when we are feeling sexual, our nipples may stand out a little more, and the areola may pucker up and get bumpy. Otherwise, during childhood our breasts are flat and smooth, and only the nipple stands out. During puberty, the breasts begin to swell and to stand out more. The nipple and areola get larger and darker in color.

Inside the Breast

In order to understand why your breasts are swelling and beginning to stand out, you have to understand what is happening beneath the skin of your breast. Illustration 10 shows the inside of a grown woman's breast. Although you can only see three of them in this picture, a woman's breast is made up of fifteen to twenty-five separate parts, called *lobes*. The lobes are like the separate sections of an orange, all packed together inside the breast. They are surrounded by a cushion of fat. Inside each lobe is a sort of tree. The leaves of these trees are called *alveoli*. When a woman has a baby, milk is made inside these leaves. The milk travels from the leaves, through the branches and trunk of the tree, which are called milk ducts, to the nipple. When a mother breastfeeds, the baby sucks on the nipple and out comes the milk.

As you begin puberty, you start to develop milk ducts under your breasts and fat tissue forms around those ducts to protect them. These milk ducts and fat

areola (ah-REE-oh-la)
alveoli (al-VEE-oh-lie)

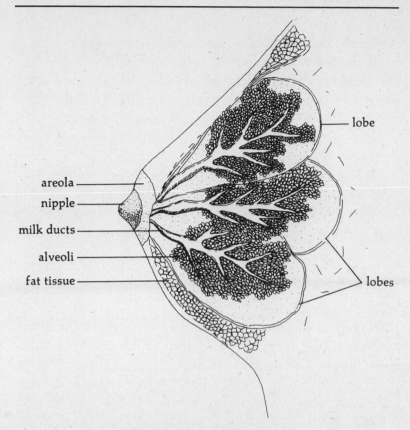

lobe

areola

nipple

milk ducts

alveoli

fat tissue

lobes

Illustration 10. Cross Section of an Adult Breast

tissue form a small mound under the nipple and areola called a *breast bud*. Your breasts are not yet ready to make milk and won't be able to do so until you have had a baby. But your body is beginning to get ready for the time when you may decide to have a baby, and this is what causes your breasts to swell and stand out.

Breast Development

No one can say for sure when a girl's breasts will start to develop. Sometimes it starts to happen when the girl is only eight and at other times not until after she is sixteen or older. Most girls begin to develop breast buds between their ninth and fourteenth birthdays. But you may not be like most girls, so you may start earlier or later than this. Starting earlier or later than most girls does not mean there is anything wrong with you. It simply means that your body is growing at its own special rate.

Doctors have divided breast growth into five different stages that are pictured in Illustration 11. You may be in one of these stages or in between one stage and another. See if you can find the stage you're closest to.

Stage 1 shows how the breasts look during childhood. The breasts are flat, and the only part that is raised is the nipple.

Stage 2 is the breast-bud stage, when the milk ducts and fat tissue form a small, buttonlike mound under each nipple and areola, making them stick out. The nipple starts to get larger. This often happens just before the breast bud starts to form. The areola gets wider, and the nipple and areola get darker in color.

In Stage 3 the breasts get rounder and fuller and begin to stand out more. The nipple may continue to get larger and the areola wider. Both may get darker in color. The breasts are usually rather cone-shaped in this stage.

Stage 4 is a stage that many, but not all, girls go through. Girls who do go through it will notice that the areola and nipple form a separate little mound so that they stick out above the rest of the breast. Illustration 12 shows a closeup of the nipple and areola in Stage 3, Stage 4, and Stage 5 so you can see the difference more clearly.

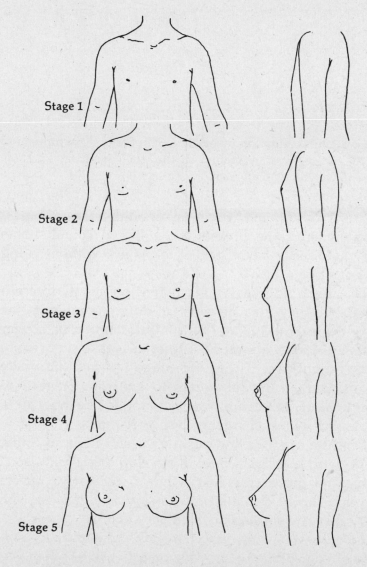

Stage 1

Stage 2

Stage 3

Stage 4

Stage 5

Illustration 11. The Five Stages of Breast Development

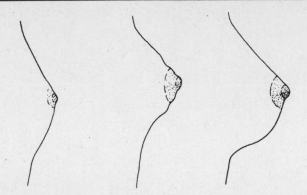

Illustration 12. Nipple in Stages 3, 4, 5. In Stage 4, the nipple and areola form a separate mound so that they stick out from the general contour of the breast.

Stage 5 shows the grown-up, or adult, stage of breast development. The breasts are full and round. Some girls go directly from Stage 3 to Stage 5 without going through Stage 4.

Not only do breasts start developing at different ages, but they also develop at different rates. Some girls begin Stage 2, and within six months or a year they are already at Stage 5. Other girls take six or more years to go from Stage 2 to Stage 5. Most girls take about four and a half years to go from Stage 2 to Stage 5, but once again, you may not be like most girls, so you may take a longer or a shorter time.

Starting early or starting late doesn't have anything to do with how fast you will develop. Some girls start early and grow very fast, while other early starters develop slowly. Some girls who start late grow slowly, but other late starters develop very quickly.

Nor does starting early or starting late have anything to do with how big your breasts will be when you are fully grown. An early starter may wind up having either large or small breasts. The same is true for late starters—they may end up with large breasts or with small ones.

Breast Development and Your First Period

Most girls have their first menstrual period while they are in Stage 4 of breast development. However, a fair number will have their period while they are only in Stage 3, and some don't have their first period until after they've reached Stage 5. A few girls will have their first period while they are in Stage 2. If you have your first period while you are only in Stage 1 (before your breasts have begun to develop), you should see a doctor. Having your period before your breasts have begun to develop doesn't necessarily mean that something's wrong, but it *may* mean that you have a problem that needs a doctor's attention.

Feelings About Developing Breasts

The mothers and daughters we talked to all had different kinds of feelings about their breasts. Some girls were really excited when their breasts started developing, like this girl who told us:

> I was so happy when my breasts started growing. First my nipples got bigger. Then my breasts started sticking out. I was so proud. I felt real grown up. I was always showing them off to my mom and my little sister.

Although many girls feel excited, they also worry about one thing or another. One girl said:

> I was really freaked out. I had these little flat bumps under my nipples, and they hurt all the time, especially if they got hit or something. They were so sore. I thought maybe something was wrong.

One or both of your breasts *may* feel tender, sore, or downright painful at times. This is perfectly normal, and it doesn't mean that anything is wrong. Although it may be a bit uncomfortable, this soreness isn't anything to worry about. It's just part of growing up.

One question that regularly comes out of my class question box is "Could a girl's breasts burst?" or, as one girl wrote, "Could a girl's boobs pop like a balloon?" Each time I get one of these questions, I always answer, "No, that can't happen," but secretly I've always wondered where in the world anyone could have gotten an idea like that. Then one day, one of the girls came up after class and explained:

> Grown-ups are always saying things like, "Oh, you're really popping out," or "You're sure bursting out all over," and sometimes my breasts feel sore, like they really are about to burst, so I wondered.

This girl made me realize how confusing the things adults say can sound to kids sometimes. If you've worried about this same thing, you can stop worrying. I can assure you that even though it may feel that way at times, your breasts won't pop or burst.

Other girls we talked to told us that they worried because both their breasts didn't develop at the same rate. One girl said:

> One of my breasts was starting to grow, and the other one was still completely flat. I was afraid that the other one would never grow, and I was only going to have one breast instead of two.

Another girl explained:

> Both of mine started growing at the same time, but one of mine was a lot bigger than the other one, and I was worried that I was going to grow up all lopsided.

It often happens that one breast develops before the other or that one seems to be growing at a much faster rate than the other. Even though one may start growing first, the other will eventually grow too. By the time a girl is fully developed, both breasts are pretty much the same size. Many grown women do notice that one breast is slightly larger than the other, but this difference in size is generally too small to be noticed by anyone other than the woman herself.

Some girls notice that tiny hairs begin to develop around the areola. One of the girls that this happened to told us:

> I started growing these little hairs around my nipple, and none of my friends did. I thought I was weird, so I plucked them out with tweezers, but they just grew back.

Although most women don't grow hairs like this, many do. It's quite normal. Plucking these hairs doesn't usually get rid of them, for most of the time they just grow back. In fact, plucking them out could cause problems, for it might start an infection that could make your breast sore, red, and painful.

"One of my nipples didn't stick out and the other did," yet another girl told us. "It sort of puckered in, and I wondered why."

This girl had what is known as an inverted nipple. One or both nipples in some girls and women sink into the areola instead of sticking out. As a girl grows older, the inverted nipple may start to stick out. Lots of women have inverted nipples. They don't cause any problems. You may have heard that women with inverted nipples can't breastfeed their babies. This is simply not true. The only time that inverted nipples might be a problem is in an adult woman when a nipple that wasn't inverted suddenly becomes inverted, or vice versa. This doesn't necessarily mean that anything is wrong, but it is something to check out with your doctor.

Some girls we talked to worried because they noticed a little fluid coming from their nipples once in awhile. This is normal. It is your body's way of keeping your ducts open. The fluid may be whitish or clear or slightly yellow or green. If there is a lot of it or if it is dark brown or has pus in it, see your doctor, for it may be a sign of an infection. (We'll talk more about inverted nipples and fluids coming out of the nipples later on when we talk about breast self-exam.)

As we said earlier, many of the girls we talked to felt excited and proud about developing breasts, but many also felt uncomfortable or embarrassed. A twenty-two-year-old told us:

> I was only in fourth grade when I started developing, and no one else was. I used to wrap one of those bandages, the kind you put on a sprained ankle, around my chest to make me flat. I kept my coat on as much as I could and wore baggy clothes all the time. Now that I'm older, I can laugh about it, but back then it wasn't funny at all.

Many of the girls and women whose breasts started developing earlier than most talked about feeling embarrassed. Girls whose breasts began to develop late often had embarrassed feelings too. One woman, now in her thirties, told us:

> I didn't start to develop until after my sixteenth birthday. Everyone, and I mean *everyone*, had breasts but me. They were all in their bras, and there I was in my undershirt. I flunked gym in high school because I wouldn't take a shower. I was too embarrassed about my flat chest. Finally, my mom bought me a padded bra. My breasts did eventually start to develop, but I really felt bad about myself for a lot of years before they did.

Another woman told us:

> I didn't start developing until I was seventeen. I thought there was something horribly wrong, like maybe I was really a man instead of a woman. Oh, and the teasing I had to endure! The boys used to call me "ironing board" because my chest was so flat.

Even girls who were neither early nor late starters feel embarrassed. As one girl put it:

> I started to develop when I was eleven, just about the same time as everyone else. I was glad that I was getting tits, but I was embarrassed, especially at school.

Our parents, our brothers and sisters, our friends, people at school may tease us about developing breasts, and this may make us feel embarrassed at times. Even strangers, people on the street, may make comments on our changing bodies. Boys or men may whistle or make sexual remarks. Sometimes this attention is flattering. As one girl explained:

> If I'm walking down the street and some guy says, "Hey, there!" or whistles or something, I feel pretty good, like he's saying, "Oh, you look good," especially if I'm with a girlfriend or a bunch of girls.

But a lot of girls and women don't like this kind of attention:

> I hate when boys stare at my breasts or whistle or yell stuff at me. It makes me feel like a piece of meat, and it makes me feel self-conscious and dumb. I mean, what can you do? Yell back at them? How would they like it if girls went down the street and stared at their crotches and yelled stuff like, "Hey, that's a really big penis you got there!" Boys do that. They say stuff like, "Hey, that's a great set of jugs!" I don't like it.

Often there isn't much you can do about this unwanted attention, beyond simply ignoring it. But it
may be helpful to talk about these experiences with
other girls so you can help each other deal with such
situations.

Bras

We get a lot of questions about when a girl should start
wearing a bra or if she even needs to wear one at all.
There are no clear-cut answers to these questions; it's
something you have to decide for yourself.

Some girls decide to wear a bra because they feel more
comfortable having some support, so their breasts don't
jiggle around when they walk, run, dance, or play
games. Others decide to wear bras because they feel
self-conscious without one. Some girls wear bras because they've heard that your breasts will eventually
begin to droop or sag if you don't wear a bra. Actually,
though, you don't need to worry about this type of
drooping unless you are fairly large-breasted and/or
you go without a bra for a number of years. One girl
in our classes had something interesting to say about
this:

> So what if your breasts droop? I mean, who says that
> breasts that don't droop are better than breasts that do?
> I don't care. I don't wear a bra and I'm not going to. I
> hate the way they feel, like I'm in a harness or some-
> thing.

We should also mention that there are many girls
who would like to wear a bra even though they aren't
very developed and don't really "need" one. One girl
who wrote to us put it this way:

I'm eleven years old . . . I'm not very big. In fact, I'm kind of flat. Do you think it is silly for me to want a bra?

When girls tell us that they're worried about seeming silly, we try to make them see that there's nothing silly about wearing a bra, no matter how "flat" you are. If the other kids or adults tease you about wearing a bra before you really "need" one, you can always say something like, "Oh, I'm just getting used to wearing one," or "I like them better than undershirts," or "I feel more comfortable this way."

Many girls have told us that they feel they'd like to start wearing a bra, but they're too embarrassed to ask their parents for one. We encourage girls who feel embarrassed about asking for a bra to go ahead and ask anyhow. Many times, parents are waiting for you to bring the topic up yourself because they don't want to embarrass you! If you feel funny about asking for a bra, you might say, "Would it be okay with you if I wore a bra?" or "When do you think I should start wearing a bra?" Or, you could write a note explaining how you feel. If your parents says something like, "Oh, don't be silly, you don't need one yet," you could say, "Well, maybe not, but I'd *like* one anyhow."

Buying a bra

Bras can be purchased at almost any store that sells women's clothing. Some clothing stores have a special lingerie (underwear) section, and the lingerie saleswoman can help you choose the size and style that's best for you.

Training bras are bras that have a flat or practically

flat cup and are made to fit girls whose breasts haven't started to develop or whose breasts are just beginning to grow. There are also one-size-fits-all bras that have cups made of elastic material that stretches to fit your shape. However, if you are very large or very small, these one-size-fits-all bras may not work for you.

In addition to training bras and one-size-fits-all bras, there are also fitted bras, which come in various sizes. The size has two parts: a number ranging from 28 to 44, which indicates the number of inches around your chest, and a letter that indicates the size of the cup. Cup sizes run from A through D or E. There are also double or triple A (AA or AAA) sizes for very small breasts, and double E (EE) for very large breasts.

To determine your proper size, first measure around your body just under your breasts, as shown in Illustration 13. Then add 5 inches to that measurement. This will give you your bra size in inches. For example, if the measurement under your breasts is 27 inches, you would add 5 inches to get 32 inches, which would be your bra size in inches.

Next, you'll need to get an idea of your cup size. Measure around the widest part of your chest, across your nipples, as shown in Illustration 13. Take this measurement and compare it to your bra size in inches (above).

If the bra size in inches is *larger* than the measurement across your nipples, you need an AAA cup size or a training bra. If the two measurements are the same, you need an AA or AAA cup. If the measurement across your nipples is 1 inch larger than your bra size, you need an A cup; if it's 2 inches larger you need a B cup; if it's 3 inches larger, you need a C cup; if it's 4 inches larger, you need a D cup; if it's 5 inches, you need an E cup. If it's 6 or more inches, you may need to buy your bra at a specialty shop where they sell larger-sized clothes.

This method of determining your cup size will give you a rough idea of your proper cup size, but it's always best to try the bra on to insure proper fit and comfort.

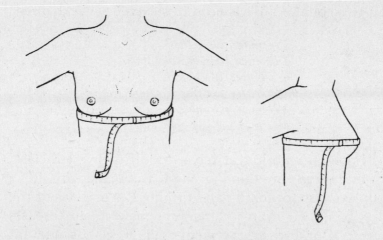

Illustration 13. Measuring for a Bra. To determine your bra size, measure yourself with a tape measure, as shown here.

You may have heard about padded bras and falsies. Padded bras have a pad of cotton or foam rubber inside the cup. When you wear a padded bra, it appears that your breasts are larger than they really are. Falsies are breast-shaped inserts that are worn inside the cup of a bra—again, to make it seem as if your breasts are larger than they actually are.

Breast Size

When I was a girl, we used to do an exercise in gym class where we'd hold our arms at shoulder level, elbows bent, and jerk our elbows back to a one-two, one-two count. While we did this exercise, we chanted:

> *We must, we must,*
> *We must increase our busts.*
> *It's better, it's better,*
> *It's better for the sweater.*
> *We may, we may,*
> *We may get big someday.*

I hope girls no longer have to do this in gym class, not that there's anything wrong with the exercise. It's a good exercise for toning and firming the muscles of the chest wall. (It won't, however, make your breasts larger. Your breasts are composed of glands and fat tissue and no amount of exercise will enlarge them. If you do this exercise a lot, the chest muscles underneath the breast will get thicker and this will make your breasts stand out more.)

No, there's nothing wrong with the exercise itself, it's the chant that went along with it—all that business about "we must increase our busts" and the emphasis on having big breasts, as if big breasts were somehow better than small ones. Breasts feel the same and can give us the same pleasurable feelings when they are stroked or touched regardless of their size. Small breasts do just as good a job of making breast milk as large ones. But with all the big-busted, glamorous women in advertisements, films, and TV shows, it's easy to get the idea that big breasts are more womanly or more sexy than small ones. But despite all the advertising, there are a great many people who find small breasts equally, if not more, attractive than large ones. And anyone who decides whether he or she likes you or not because of the size of your breasts probably isn't a person worth knowing anyhow.

Still, we do live in a country that has a hang-up about breasts. Some women with small breasts who feel self-conscious may have a difficult time, which is why there are padded bras and falsies and operations to enlarge breasts. If padded bras or falsies sound like the right choice for you, you can find them in the bra section of any department store and the salesclerk will help fit you. Breast size can be a problem for large-breasted women too. Some women have such large breasts that it affects their posture and causes back pains. Having tremendously big breasts can be embarrassing too. If you have this problem, you should know that there are also operations to reduce breasts to a more comfortable size. Operations to reduce or enlarge breasts can't be done, however, until you are fully grown because your breasts are still developing and the operation could interfere with normal development.

Regardless of whether your breasts are large or small or medium-size, it's important that you learn how to practice breast self-exam.

Breast Self-Exam

Breast self-exam means examining your breasts to see if there are any lumps or other irregularities that might be signs of breast cancer.

Not all breast lumps are signs of cancer. In fact, the

vast majority of lumps that women find in their breasts are *not* cancerous. But since cancer can appear as a small lump in the breast, it is important to examine your breasts and have a doctor check any lumps you do find to rule out the possibility of breast cancer.

One out of every eleven women in this country gets breast cancer. In some cases, breast cancer can be cured by removing the lump. Other times, it is necessary to remove the whole breast. Sometimes, breast cancer can't be cured and the woman dies. If a woman discovers her breast cancer while the lump is small, she has a much better chance of being cured. That's why breast self-exam is so important. If a woman feels her breasts regularly, once a month, she has a better chance of being able to find the lump right away, before the cancer is so serious that it can't be cured.

Actually, breast exam is not very important for teenagers because teenagers don't, as a rule, get breast cancer. (There have been a few young women who've had breast cancer, but it's very rare.) Many doctors tell women to start examining their breasts after they've reached their twenty-fifth birthdays, since breast cancer is rare before the age of twenty-five.

We suggest that young women start examining their breasts as soon as they have had their first menstrual periods. We think this is a good idea for two reasons. First of all, it gets you started, while you're young, on what should become a lifelong habit. But perhaps more importantly, if you're examining your breasts regularly, it might get your mom, your older sisters, or other women you may live with to do it too. Far too many women neglect this live-saving measure. Maybe your doing it will set an example for them. Why don't you and your mom or another adult woman try practicing breast exam, which is described below, together?

Breast exam should be done about once a month. The best time is right after your menstrual period is over. Some women's breasts tend to be a little lumpy before or during their menstrual periods because the ducts and tissues of the breast swell a bit. If you are one of these women, you will find that your breasts are less lumpy just after your period, so it will be easier to do the exam at that time.

Breast exam should be done when you are relaxed and are not feeling rushed. The exam consists of two parts: 1) looking at your breasts, and 2) feeling them.

PART ONE: LOOKING (ILLUSTRATION 14)

To begin, stand in front of a well-lighted mirror with your arms down at your sides and take a good look at your breasts from the front and from each side. Look to see if there are any depressions, bulges, moles, dimples, dark or red areas, swellings, sores, or areas of skin with a rough or orange peel-like texture. Check the nipple and areola as well as the skin of the breast. If you have any of these problems, keep an eye on them and if they're not gone in a couple of weeks, see a doctor. At your age, these problems aren't likely to be signs of cancer, but you may have a noncancerous problem in your breast that needs attention.

Next, put your hands on your hips and press inward and down so that the muscles of your upper chest tighten. Check to see if the muscles contract about the same amount or if any bulging or dimpling shows up on your breasts when you've got your muscles tight like this. Sometimes, a lump that isn't noticeable in the first position will become obvious only when you tighten. While your hands are still on your hips, rotate to each side, looking for the same things.

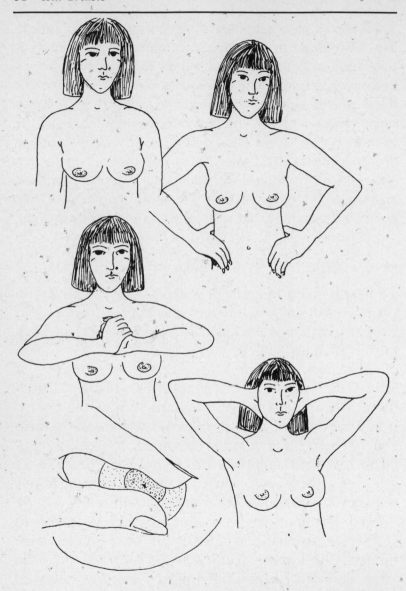

Illustration 14. Breast Self-Exam, Part One: Looking. Stand in front of a mirror and inspect your breasts in each of the four positions shown here. Finally, squeeze each nipple for signs of discharge.

Now put your arms in front of your chest at about heart level, press your palms together, and check for uneven muscle contraction, bulges, or dimpling. Check each side of your breasts. If your breasts are large or hang down, you may have to lift each breast to check the underside.

Next raise your arms, bend your elbows, and place your hands behind your head. Once again, check from the front and from both sides for any signs of dimpling or bulging that might indicate a lump or thickening inside the breast.

To finish the first part of the exam, gently squeeze each nipple to see if you can get any fluid to come out. Fluid from the nipple is not necessarily a sign that something is wrong. But if there is a lot of it or if it is dark in color or full of pus, see a doctor.

PART TWO: FEELING (ILLUSTRATION 15)

This part is done lying down because when you lie down your breasts spread out and it will be easier to feel for lumps. Lotion or oil will make your fingers more sensitive.

To begin, bend one arm and place your hand behind your head. Use the fatty pads of your fingers rather than your fingertips, and starting on the outside of your breast, using a circular motion, carefully feel each breast. Press all the way down to the chest wall. Also feel the upper part of your chest and under your armpit. Repeat the process on the other side.

What you are looking, or rather, feeling for, is any lump or thickening in the breast, the chest, or under the armpits. This sounds pretty simple, but it can be tricky. For one thing, it's kind of like feeling for a

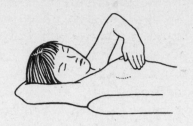

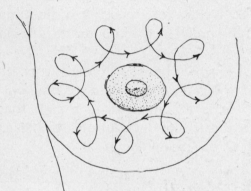

Illustration 15. Breast Self-Exam, Part Two: Feeling. Lie down with one hand behind your head. With your other hand, start on the outside of your breast and, using a circular motion, feel the entire breast. Repeat on the opposite breast.

marble in a bag filled with Jello. Every time you press near it, the lump moves away. You may have to use two hands now and then to support your breast in order to get a good feel. It's also hard because most women have rather bumpy or even lumpy breasts. It's easy to mistake the ducts, the ribs, the breastbone, or the underlying muscles for lumps. Once you have been doing it for a while, though, you'll be able to tell the difference between the normal lumps and bumps and any abnormal ones.

If you find any lumps, thickening, red spots, bulges, or unusual fluid from your nipples, or if a nipple suddenly becomes inverted (or if an inverted nipple suddenly begins to stick out), *don't panic.* Remember, breast cancer in young women is very, very rare. But there are other, noncancerous conditions that can affect young girls' breasts. So, if your symptoms last more than two weeks, get them checked out.

CHAPTER 5

Changes in the Vulva

The genital organs on the outside of your body, which are sometimes referred to as the vulva, also change as you go through puberty. The various parts of the vulva are easy to see if you hold a mirror between your legs as the girl in Illustration 16 is doing. The other drawings in Illustration 16 show how the vulva looks in a young girl, in a young woman going through puberty, and in a grown woman.

The easiest way to learn about these organs and how they change during puberty is to use a mirror and compare your own body to these drawings. You probably won't look exactly like any of these drawings because each person's body is a little bit different. But if you looked at a drawing of a person's face with eyes, a nose, a mouth, and so on, you could easily find the eyes, nose, or mouth on your own face, even if the drawing didn't look *exactly* like your own face. In the

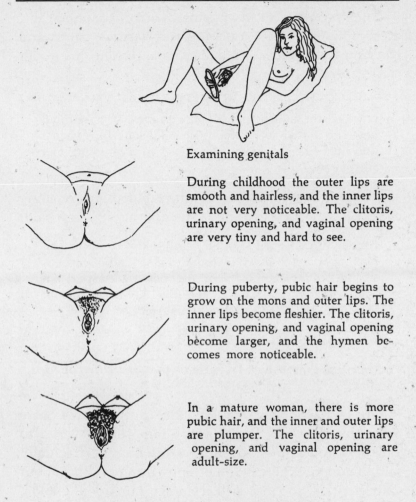

Examining genitals

During childhood the outer lips are smooth and hairless, and the inner lips are not very noticeable. The clitoris, urinary opening, and vaginal opening are very tiny and hard to see.

During puberty, pubic hair begins to grow on the mons and outer lips. The inner lips become fleshier. The clitoris, urinary opening, and vaginal opening become larger, and the hymen becomes more noticeable.

In a mature woman, there is more pubic hair, and the inner and outer lips are plumper. The clitoris, urinary opening, and vaginal opening are adult-size.

Illustration 16. Examining the Genitals

same way, you can look at a drawing of a vulva and find the various parts on your own vulva. Of course, we're a lot more used to looking at faces than vulvas, but with a little practice, you can learn to see the features of your vulva as plainly as you can see the nose on your face.

Some people think that using a mirror to look at this area of their bodies, touching the various parts, and learning their names is a dandy idea. As one girl in our class said:

> Oh, I've looked at myself there lots of times. My mom got a mirror and showed me how to look at myself and how she looked so I'd know what I'll look like when I grow up. She taught me the names of everything and all that stuff.

Other girls don't feel as comfortable about touching or looking at their genitals. One girl in our class said:

> I thought it sounded kind of weird, taking a mirror and looking at myself down there, but I was kind of curious, so I locked my bedroom door and took a good look. I'm glad I did, 'cause it made me feel like I know more about myself, like it wasn't such a big mystery.

Still another girl said:

> Ugh, that's disgusting. I'd never do that. It's yucky down there.

This girl had been taught that her genitals were dirty and ugly and that it was shameful or wrong to look at or touch them. Even if no one has never actually said to you that there is something wrong or dirty about your genitals, you may still feel uncertain about exploring them. People don't talk about genital organs very much, and as we all know, if something is too terrible to talk about, then it's probably really terrible!

But there is nothing terrible or wrong about this area of your body. People feel uncomfortable because it is a sexual part of the body, and people often feel uncomfortable about anything that has to do with sex. Some people get the idea that this part of the body is dirty because the openings through which urine and feces leave our bodies are located here. Actually, this area of our bodies isn't any dirtier than, say, the inside of our mouths. (In fact, our mouths have more germs than this area of our bodies.)

In the following pages, we'll take you on a guided tour of the vulva and explain how your genitals change during puberty. If you don't feel comfortable about touching or looking at your genitals, that's fine. Just read these pages and look at the pictures. We wouldn't want you to do anything you don't feel okay doing. If you'd like to, though, we think you'll find it helpful to keep a mirror handy so you can look at yourself as you read about these parts of your body. You may want to do this all by yourself, with a friend, or with your mom. Do whatever feels most comfortable for you.

The Mons

We'll start our tour at the top of the vulva, at the mons. As you may remember, the mons is a pad of fat tissue that covers the pubic bone. It is here, on the mons, that pubic hair begins to grow during puberty, and in grown women the mons is covered with curly pubic hair.

In addition to sprouting hair, the mons also gets fleshier during puberty so that it sticks out more. This is because the fat pad over the pubic bone is getting thicker.

The Outer Lips

As you move down along the mons, you will see that it divides into two separate flaps, or folds, of skin. As we told you earlier, these are the outer lips, or the labia majora. *Labia* is a Latin word meaning lips and *majora* means major or big, so they are sometimes called the "major lips" or "big lips."

In a young girl, the outer lips may be hairless, or they may have a few light-colored hairs. During puberty, pubic hair begins to grow on the outer lips.

In young girls, the lips are often separated. There may be space between them, so they may not actually touch each other. During puberty, the lips get fleshier and they often begin to touch. In grown women, the lips generally touch, but some women find that after they've had a baby, the lips are slightly separated again. In very old women, the lips get thinner, less fleshy, and may become separated again.

The lips are usually smooth in a young girl, but during puberty, they may get sort of wrinkly. In grown women, they tend to be wrinkly. Many women find that when they are old and gray, the lips get smooth again.

The outer lips help protect the area underneath. The underside of the lips usually is hairless, both in young girls and in grown women. In girls, the underside of the lips is smooth, but as you go through puberty, you may notice small, slightly raised bumps dotting the skin on the underside of the lips. These are oil glands. They make a small amount of oil that keeps the area moist so that it doesn't get irritated. Once you start puberty, you may notice a slight feeling of wetness in this area because of this oil. You may also notice a change in the way this area of your body smells. Again, this is because of the oil made by these glands.

During childhood, this area may be light pink to red to brownish-black in color, depending on your skin tone. The color is apt to change during puberty, getting either lighter or darker.

The Inner Lips

If you separate the outer lips, you will see two ridges, or folds, of skin called the *labia minora*, the minor lips, or the little lips. During childhood, the inner lips may not be very noticeable, but during puberty, they grow and become more noticeable. Like the outer lips, they protect the area between them, and they too tend to change color and get more wrinkly during puberty.

As you can see in Illustration 17, the labia look different in different women. In most women, the inner lips are smaller than the outer lips, but in some women, the inner lips protrude beyond the outer lips. The inner lips are usually about the same size, but some women notice that one is larger than the other.

The inner lips are hairless in both girls and grown women. They tend to be more moist as we grow older because they too have oil glands that begin producing more oil during puberty.

The Clitoris

If you follow the inner lips up toward the mons, you will see that they join together at the top. In the area where the inner lips join together lies the tip of the clitoris, in slang terms, the "clit." In grown women, the clitoris is about the size of the eraser on the end of a pencil. The way in which the inner lips join together is not the same in all women. In some women, the inner lips come together forming a sort of hood that covers the clitoris. In other women, the clitoris sticks all or part

minora (mi-NOR-ah)

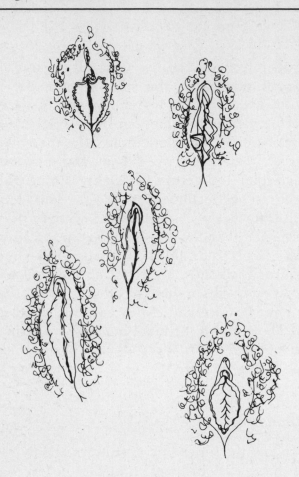

Illustration 17 . The Labia. The inner lips look different in different women.

of the way out from the folds of the hood formed by the inner lips. When we are feeling sexual, the clitoris tends to swell and get a little larger for a while. It also grows permanently larger during puberty.

You may have to pull back the hood formed by the inner lips in order to see the clitoris; even then you can only see the tip of the clitoris. The rest of the clitoris lies buried under the skin. If you press down on the skin above the clitoris, you may be able to feel a rubbery cord under the skin. This is the shaft of the clitoris.

Masturbation

The clitoris and its shaft—in fact, this whole area of your body—is very sensitive. When you touch it, you may get an excited, tingly kind of feeling. Touching, rubbing, stroking, or squeezing this area of your body so that you will have these feelings is called *masturbating* or *masturbation*. There are also lots of slang words for masturbation, such as "jerking off," "playing with yourself," or "jacking off."

Sometimes when people masturbate, they get so excited that they have a shivery feeling that is called an *orgasm*. Having an orgasm is also called "coming" or "climaxing." It's hard to explain exactly what an orgasm feels like, and orgasms probably feel different to different people, but most people agree that it is a good feeling.

Not everyone masturbates, but many if not most of us do at some time or other in our lives. Some women start masturbating when they are children and continue to do so all their lives. Some start during puberty; others don't start until they are grown women. Still others never masturbate. It's normal if you do it and normal if you don't.

Many men and boys also masturbate. They do so by touching or stroking their penises. (This is explained more fully in Chapter 8, Puberty in Boys.)

Some people think that once a person starts having

masturbating (MASS-tur-bait-ing)
masturbation (MASS-tur-bay-shun)
orgasm (or-GAZ-um)
climaxing (KLY-max-ing)

sexual intercourse or gets married, that person no longer masturbates. This isn't true. People who have sex regularly often continue to masturbate either alone or with their sexual partner.

You may have heard all sorts of strange things about masturbation. People used to think that masturbation would make you insane or make you go blind or turn you into a moron. Obviously, these things aren't true or there would be an awful lot of insane, blind morons around. You may have heard that masturbation will cause you to grow hair on the palms of your hands, pimples on your face, warts on your fingers, or other strange things. Again, none of this is true. You may have heard that masturbation will make you enjoy sex with another person less; this is also not true. Actually, masturbating can be a way of rehearsing for your adult sex life. Most sex experts feel that by learning how to give yourself pleasure sexually, you are taking the first step in learning how to have sexual pleasure with someone else.

One question that frequently comes up in my classes is whether or not masturbating "too much" can hurt you in some way. The answer is no. Nothing bad will happen to your body regardless of how much you masturbate; masturbation is not physically harmful in any way. About the only thing that can happen is that your genitals might get a little sore if you are masturbating and rubbing them a whole lot. Some people masturbate every day. Some masturbate many times in one day. Others only rarely masturbate, and still others never do. Remember, it's normal if you do it and normal if you don't.

Some people like to imagine things that make them feel more excited when they are masturbating. Imagining or pretending that something is happening is called

daydreaming or fantasizing. We daydream and fanta-
size about all sorts of things. When our daydreams are
about sexual things, we call them sexual fantasies. Almost everyone has sexual fantasies. Fantasies can be a
rich and varied way of experimenting with your sexual
self. So our advice is: relax and enjoy them.

For some people, having sexual fantasies and/or
masturbating is in conflict with their religious or moral
beliefs. These people feel that a person shouldn't allow
himself or herself to have such fantasies or to masturbate. For other people, having sexual fantasies and masturbation is not in conflict with their religious or moral
beliefs, and these people think it's perfectly okay for a
person to do these things. Personally, we tend to go
along with this viewpoint, and we think it's fine for a
person to do these things. But, if doing these things is
in conflict with your beliefs, then you can decide not
to do them. In any case, you should know that masturbation is not physically harmful in any way.

But, let's leave the topic of masturbation and sexual
fantasies and get back to the guided tour of your body.

The Urinary Opening

If you move down your clitoris in a straight line, you
will come to the urinary opening. *Urinary* comes from
the word *urine*. Urine is made inside our bodies. The
food we eat and drink is broken down inside of us so
that our bodies can use it. Not everything we eat and
drink can be used by our bodies. After foods are
broken down and used, some of the leftovers are in the
form of the clear, yellowish, waterlike liquid called
urine. The urine collects in an organ inside our bodies
called the *bladder*. The bladder is like a balloon or bag.
It has a small tube at the bottom, which leads to the

outside of our bodies. The urinary opening is the out-side end of this tube. When our bladder is full, we press down, the tube opens up, and the urine from the bladder runs down the tube and out through the urinary opening.

It may be difficult for you to see exactly where the urinary opening is. If you start at the clitoris and move downward in a straight line, the first dimpled area you come to is the urinary opening. It may look like an upside down V. During puberty, the urinary opening becomes more noticeable than it is during childhood.

If you don't stay on a straight line down from the clitoris, you may mistake the urinary opening for one of the two tiny glands also located in this area. The openings to these glands are two little slits on either side of the urinary opening. Like the oil glands on the inner and outer lips, these glands make a small amount of oil that keeps this area moist. Some women have such tiny openings to these glands that they can't be seen; others have larger ones that can be mistaken for the urinary opening.

The Vaginal Opening

Now that you know where the urinary opening is, you'll be able to find the vaginal opening. As we ex-plained earlier, the vagina is up inside your body, so you won't be able to see the vagina itself, but you will be able to find the opening to the vagina. If you move down from the urinary opening—again, in a straight line—you'll come to the vaginal opening.

Pictures of the vaginal opening are sometimes con-

bladder (BLAD-er)

fusing since they make it look as if the vaginal opening
is a dark, gaping hole. It's not. The vagina itself is like
a pouch. In young girls, it's not very big. During puberty, it starts to grow, but even in adult women, it's
only three to five inches long. But the vagina is like
a balloon, and it can expand to many times its size. It
has to be able to expand like this so a man's penis can
fit in there during sexual intercourse. Also, when a
woman has a baby, the baby travels through the vagina
on its way out of the mother's body.

Most of the time, though, the sides of the vagina
touch each other. If you were to look into the opening
of a collapsed balloon, you wouldn't see an empty
space. You'd see the collapsed sides of the balloon all
folded up and touching each other. The same is true of
the vagina: When you look into the vaginal opening,
you don't see a hole, you see the fleshy walls of the
vagina up against each other.

The Hymen

The vaginal opening may be partly covered by a thin
piece of skin just inside the opening called the *hymen*.
Other names for the hymen are "cherry" or "maiden-
head." The hymen looks different in different women.
It may just be a thin fringe of skin around the edges
of the vaginal opening, or it may stretch all or part way
across the opening and have one or more holes in it.
Illustration 18 shows just a few of the ways the hymen
may look.

In young girls, the hymen may not be very noticeable. During puberty, it usually gets thicker and more

hymen (HI-men)

rigid and more noticeable. But not all girls have a noticeable hymen. A few are born without one. Others have such small ones that it's hard to see them. Also, it is possible for a girl to break or stretch her hymen during vigorous exercise (such as horseback riding or doing gymnastics), though this is rare.

As strange as it might seem, some people used to think that this tiny little piece of skin was *very, very* important. People thought that all women had the kind of hymens that only have a few holes and that stretch all the way across the vaginal opening. They thought that the only reason a woman wouldn't have a noticeable hymen was because it had been stretched or torn by a man's penis during sexual intercourse. Today we know this isn't true, and that having a noticeable hymen or one that has not been stretched or torn doesn't necessarily have anything to do with whether or not a woman has had sex with a man. (In fact, some women

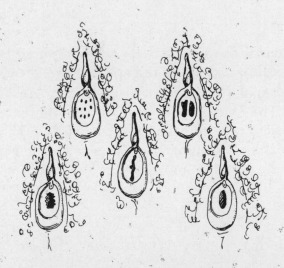

Illustration 18. The Hymen. The hymen may have one or two large openings or several small ones.

have sex with men without their hymens stretching or tearing at all.)

But in the old days, people thought that if a woman didn't have an untorn, unstretched hymen across her entire vaginal opening with only small holes in it, this meant that she had already had sex with a man and was not a virgin (a virgin is a woman who has never had sexual intercourse). People also thought that it was important that a woman be a virgin when she married. Of course, many people still feel this way, but back then a woman who was not a virgin when she got married could get into a lot of trouble. In some countries, a woman could even be put to death if she wasn't a virgin when she married. In other countries, young women were examined before marriage to see if they had a hymen. If they didn't, the marriage could be called off. In still other countries, a bride was supposed to hang her bedsheets out the window the morning after her wedding night. Since her wedding night was the first time she was supposed to have sex, and since people thought the hymen would break and bleed only in sexual intercourse, the bride's bedsheets were supposed to have blood on them as proof to everyone that she had been a virgin before her wedding night.

You can imagine the problems all this fuss about the hymen made for those women who were born without hymens, for those whose hymens had been stretched or torn during childhood, or for those whose hymens simply weren't very noticeable. Some were killed and others never married or lived their lives in disgrace. Not only that, but some women's hymens don't bleed very much when they are stretched or torn. So, even those brides who were lucky enough to have hymens

virgin (VUR-gin)

of the approved kind might not have had any blood on their wedding sheets. History is full of stories of clever brides who took a bit of animal's blood and poured it on the sheets to fool everyone. Still, it seems an awful lot of fuss about what is only a thin piece of skin.

People have, for the most part, changed their attitudes about the hymen. But, in some parts of the world, these old ideas still persist, and you may have heard some of them. If so, just ignore them. The appearance of your hymen doesn't necessarily have anything to do with whether or not you are a virgin, and you can't tell just by looking. In fact, most doctors can't tell either. It takes a specially trained doctor and even these doctors may need to use a microscope in order to tell.

When your hymen is stretched or torn—whether it's during sex or while you're doing gymnastics or riding a horse or whatever—it may bleed a little, a whole lot, or not at all. It may hurt a little, a whole lot, or not at all. If it does hurt a lot or bleed a whole lot, you should, of course, see your doctor. But only rarely does a hymen bleed or hurt so badly that a doctor's care is needed; for most women it's just not a problem.

The Anus

Although it is not really a sex organ, there is another opening in this area of the body called the *anus*. You have probably heard some of the slang terms like "asshole," "butthole," or "poophole" that are also used to refer to this opening.

If you continue moving down from the vaginal opening, you'll come to the anus. It is the outside opening to the bowels, which are long, hollow tubes that are

intestines (in-TES-tins)

coiled up inside of the body. The bowels are also called the *small intestines*.

Remember when we talked about how the food we take into our bodies is broken down and how urine is part of what is left over? Well, in addition to the watery urine, there are also more solid leftovers, which are called *feces*. People sometimes use slang words like "shit" or "poop" to refer to feces. The feces travel through the bowels and when we go to the bathroom and have a bowel movement, the feces come out through the anus.

The skin around the anus, just like the skin of the labia, may change color during puberty, getting a little darker. Pubic hair may also start to grow around the anus during puberty.

This completes the tour of the sex organs on the outside of your body. In the next chapter we will look at the inside of your body and still more changes that take place during puberty.

feces (FEE-sees)

CHAPTER 6

Changes in the Reproductive Organs

The changes occurring outside your body during puberty—the breast buds, the pubic hair, the changes in your vulva—happen because other, even more dramatic changes are taking place on the inside. In order to understand puberty and menstruation, you have to have some idea of what's going on inside you.

The Reproductive Organs

Just as we have sex organs on the outside of our bodies, so we have sex organs on the inside. The sex organs inside of our bodies are called reproductive organs because they are involved in the process of reproducing, that is, in having babies. Illustration 19 shows a side view of the reproductive organs—the vagina, uterus, tubes, and ovaries—in a young girl and in a grown woman. As you can see from these drawings, our re-cross section of reproductive organs in young girl

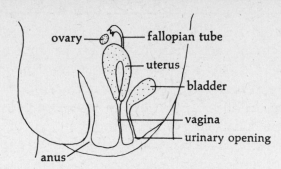

ovary — fallopian tube
uterus
bladder
vagina
urinary opening
anus

cross section of reproductive organs in older woman

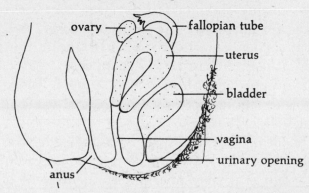

ovary — fallopian tube
uterus
bladder
vagina
urinary opening
anus

Illustration 19. Cross Section of Reproductive Organs. Our reproductive organs change as we get older. They grow larger and also change positions as they grow. Note that the uterus is almost vertical in a young girl, but is tilted forward in a woman.

productive organs also change as we get older. In this chapter we'll be talking about the changes that take place in these organs during puberty.

The Vagina

In the last chapter, you learned where the opening to your vagina is located. As we explained, the vagina itself is inside the body. The vagina is rather like a pouch tucked up inside us, which is very elastic or stretchy so that a man's penis can fit inside it during sexual intercourse. It is so stretchable that it can expand to allow a baby to pass from the uterus and through the vagina during childbirth. Most of the time, though, the vagina is like a collapsed balloon without any air in it, and the inside walls of the vagina are all folded up and touching each other.

The vagina, like the other organs in our bodies, grows during childhood. And, like other parts of our bodies, it undergoes a growth spurt during puberty, so that it suddenly starts becoming longer until it reaches its adult length of three to five inches.

If you put your finger up inside your vagina, you'll be able to feel the soft, squishy vaginal walls all folded up against each other.

The idea of putting your finger up inside your vagina might seem a little weird. Many girls, and women too, are afraid that they might hurt themselves or injure themselves in some way by doing this. But there's nothing mysterious or breakable in there. You could no more injure yourself by putting a finger inside your vagina than you could by putting a finger inside your mouth. However, your vaginal opening and hymen may be rather small and tight, so it's possible that it might feel a bit uncomfortable to you, especially if you are feeling a bit nervous about exploring yourself in this way. There's a simple rule to follow here: If it hurts too much, don't do it. Using some K-Y Jelly might help make it easier, but don't use body lotions or other skin creams that have perfumes and chemicals added, as they could be irritating. If the opening to your vagina is so tight and small that it's hard to get your finger in there, you might want to slowly stretch the opening over a period of a few weeks or months. Running your

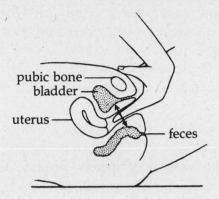

pubic bone
bladder
uterus
feces

Illustration 20. The Vagina. If you press up toward the mons, you may feel the pubic bone and the urethra, the tube through which urine travels from the bladder. If you press down, you may feel lumps of feces in the lower bowel.

finger around the opening from time to time (while you're taking a hot bath is a good time) will help stretch it.

If you press upward, just inside the vaginal opening you'll feel a bone covered by a soft bulge of tissue. It may feel rather sensitive, for underneath this bulge lies the urethra, the tube that runs from the bottom of the bladder to the outside of your body. Pressing upward in this manner may give you the feeling that you have to urinate because the bladder lies quite near the vagina, and any pressure on the bladder can give you the feeling that you have to pee (see Illustration 20).

If you press down on the vaginal walls, you may feel some lumps. This is because the lower part of your

urethra (you-REE-thra)

bowels lie just under the vagina, so you may be able to feel lumps of feces in the lower bowel.

If you slide your fingers more deeply into the vagina and press on the vaginal walls, you may notice that only about the first third of the vagina is very sensitive to your touch. The upper portion of the vagina is not as sensitive because it has fewer nerve endings.

The Cervix

At the top of the vagina, you may be able to feel a firm, round knob. This is the *cervix*, the lower part of the uterus that protrudes into the vagina (see Illustration 21). Like the vagina, the cervix grows larger during puberty. In grown women, it is about one to two inches in diameter.

cervix (SIR-vicks)

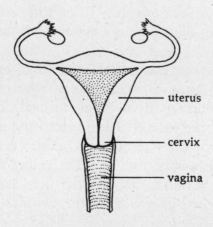

uterus

cervix

vagina

Illustration 21. The Cervix. The cervix is the lower portion of the uterus that protrudes into the vagina.

It is not always easy to feel the cervix, since it is at the top of the vagina, but if you bear down as if you were making a bowel movement you should be able to feel it. It feels rather firm, like the tip of your nose. You may be able to feel a small depression or hole in the center of the cervix. This is the opening to the cervical canal, the tunnel that leads from the vagina into the uterus. This opening is called the *os*. It is no bigger around than the head of a kitchen match. Sperm pass through the os on their way to meet the ova. Menstrual blood passes through here when you are having your period. When a woman is having a baby, the cervical canal, like the vagina, stretches so the baby can pass through.

Your cervix and the walls of your vagina may feel wet, especially when you are sexually excited, for there are glands in here that make fluids and mucus that lubricate the vagina when we are sexually excited. Even if you are not feeling sexually excited, your cervix and vagina may feel rather wet. Like the skin on the outside of your body, the skin on the inside of the vagina is continually shedding old, dead cells. During puberty, the vaginal walls begin to shed cells at a faster rate than during childhood, and the cervix and vagina begin to make a small amount of mucus and fluid to wash these cells away. A year or two (or even more) before your first menstrual period, you may start to notice a clear or milky-white, watery discharge from your vagina. It may leaves a yellowish stain on your underpants when it dries. This discharge is made up of dead cells, mucus, and fluid. This discharge is perfectly normal, just another one of the signs that puberty is beginning.

cervical (SIR-vick-ul)
os (OSZ)

If, however, the discharge has a strong, offensive odor, causes itching or redness on your vulva, or is grayish, greenish, or yellowish in color, then you may have an infection in your vagina. Such infections are not usually serious, but you should see a doctor so you can get them cleared up. (For more information, see pages 114 to 116 and 194 to 197.)

The Ovaries

The ovaries also get larger during puberty, but there is an even more dramatic change that takes place in the ovaries: It is during puberty that one of your ovaries will produce its first ripe ovum.

Unlike a male, who constantly makes a new supply of sperm in his body, a female is born with all the ova she will ever have. There are hundreds of thousands of ova in a girl's ovaries, but only eight or nine hundred of them will ever fully ripen.

The ripening process begins in the brain. When a girl is about eight years old, a part of her brain called the *pituitary* begins to send out substances called *hormones*. Hormones are made in one part of our bodies and travel to another part to act upon an organ there so that it develops or behaves in a particular way. Our bodies make hundreds of hormones. You could go crazy just trying to remember all their names. But in this book, we'll only bother with the hormones that are important in reproduction and puberty.

One of the hormones made by the pituitary during puberty is *FSH*, which is short for "follicle stimulating

pituitary (pih-TWO-eh-tear-ee)
hormones (HOR-moans)

hormone." During puberty, the FSH from the pituitary starts to get into the bloodstream and travels to the ovaries. It travels deep inside of the ovary where the tiny ova lie. Each ovum is encased in a tiny sac called a *follicle*. The follicle stimulating hormone, as its name implies, stimulates some of the follicles and their ova to grow and develop. It also causes the follicles to make yet another hormone called *estrogen* (see Illustration 22).

As a girl is going through puberty, her pituitary makes increasing amounts of FSH, which causes the follicles in the ovaries to make more and more estrogen. The estrogen also gets into the bloodstream and travels to other parts of the body. It is estrogen that causes many of the changes we notice during puberty. For example, estrogen travels to our breasts and causes the milk ducts and fat tissue to develop so that our breasts begin to swell and stand out. It causes fat tissue to develop on our hips, thighs, and buttocks, giving us a more curvy, womanly shape. Estrogen also causes pubic and other body hair to grow.

As the follicles in the ovary are developing and making increasing amounts of estrogen, they are also traveling toward the surface of the ovary. When they reach the surface, they press on the outer skin of the ovary, forming tiny bubbles that look like blisters.

Finally, when a girl is making a sufficient amount of estrogen, her pituitary gland slows down its production of FSH for a while and starts making another hormone called *LH*, or "luteinizing hormone." The LH travels to the ovary and causes one of the tiny bubbles on the

follicle (FOL-eh-kul)
estrogen (ES-tro-jen)
luteinizing (LOOT-in-eyes-ing)

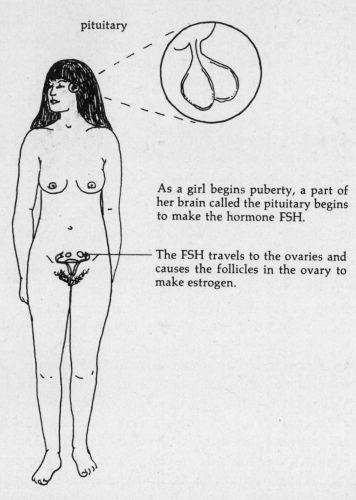

pituitary

As a girl begins puberty, a part of her brain called the pituitary begins to make the hormone FSH.

The FSH travels to the ovaries and causes the follicles in the ovary to make estrogen.

Illustration 22. Hormones. The estrogen that a girl's ovaries begin to make during puberty travels throughout her body, causing many changes, including the growth of pubic hair, swelling of the breasts, and development of fat tissue around her hips.

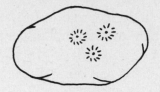

FSH from the pituitary causes some of the follicles in the ovary to develop and to make estrogen.

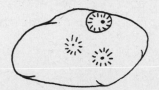

As more and more FSH reaches the ovaries, the follicles make increasing amounts of estrogen and move toward the surface of the ovary.

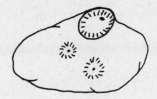

One of the follicles reaches the surface and presses on the outer skin of the ovary, forming a bubble.

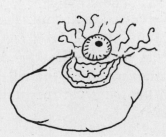

When a girl is making enough estrogen, the pituitary slows down its production of FSH and makes LH. The LH travels to the ovary, causing the follicle to burst and release its tiny ovum.

Illustration 23. Ovulation

surface of the ovary to pop, and the ripe ovum bursts off the ovary. *Ovulation* is what we call this process of the ovum popping off the ovary (see Illustration 23).

ovulation (ahv-u-LAY-shun)

Although some girls feel a slight twinge or a dull ache or even a strong pain when ovulation happens, most of us never feel the ovum popping off. A girl may ovulate for the first time when she is as young as eight or she may not ovulate until she is sixteen or older.

After ovulation, the fringed ends of the fallopian tube reach out to grasp the ovum and draw it into the tube.

The Fallopian Tubes

The fallopian tubes, through which ova travel on their way to the uterus, also grow longer and wider during puberty. But even in grown women, they are no thicker around than a strand of spaghetti. By the time we are grown women, each tube is about four inches long. The insides of the fallopian tubes are lined with tiny hairs, called *cilia*, which are attached to the muscles of the walls of the tubes. These muscles can contract and release, causing the tiny cilia to wave back and forth. It is this back-and-forth movement of the cilia that moves the ripe ovum down the length of the tube and into the uterus (see Illustration 24).

The Uterus

Like the other reproductive organs, the uterus also changes as we go through puberty. It too grows larger, but even in grown women it is only about the size of a clenched fist. The drawings in Illustration 25 show the approximate sizes of the uterus and ovaries in a typical eleven-year-old girl and in a grown woman. Try tracing them, cutting

cilia (SIL-ee-uh)

them out, and holding them up to your own body. Doing this will help you to understand the size and location of these organs and how they change as you go through puberty.

As you can see from Illustration 19 at the beginning of this chapter, the uterus not only grows larger, it also changes position during puberty. In a young girl, the uterus is in an upright, almost vertical position, but as she grows older, it begins to lean forward, so it is tilted toward the bladder. This doesn't happen to all of us. Some women have what is called a tipped uterus (see Illustration 26), which means that the uterus has remained in its nearly upright position or has tipped in the other direction. It was once thought that having a tipped uterus might make it difficult for a woman to have a baby. All manner of backaches and problems were blamed on the tipped uterus. Doctors even performed operations to tip the uterus forward. We now

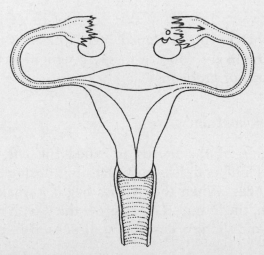

Illustration 24. The Ovum. The ovum travels through the lopian tube to the uterus.

cut along dotted lines

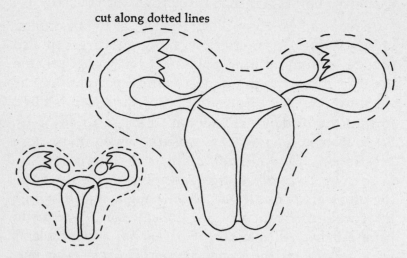

Illustration 25. The Uterus and Ovaries. Approximate drawings of uterus, fallopian tubes, and ovaries in a typical eleven-year-old girl and a grown woman.

know that having a tipped uterus has nothing to do with how likely you are to get pregnant or with any other sorts of problems.

The Endometrium

The lining of the uterus is called the *endometrium*. During childhood, it is very thin, but during puberty it too changes. When the ovaries begin to make enough estrogen, the lining starts to grow thick with new blood vessels and spongy, cushioning tissues. By the time the

endometrium (en-doe-MEE-tree-um)

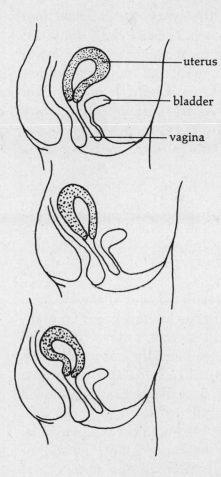

uterus

bladder

vagina

In most grown women, the uterus leans forward, toward the bladder.

But in some women, the uterus is in a more upright, vertical position.

In other women, the uterus is tipped backward, tilted away from the bladder.

Illustration 26. Tipped Uterus

LH from the pituitary has caused the first ripe egg to pop off the ovary, the endometrium has doubled in thickness and is rich with blood.

After the ovum pops off the ovary, the endometrium undergoes yet another change. The LH from the pituitary that caused the follicle on the surface of the ovary to burst also causes the remnants of the burst follicle to turn a bright yellow color. The bright yellow leftover pieces of the burst follicle on the surface of the ovary are called the *corpus luteum*, from the Latin words *corpus*, meaning "body," and *luteum*, meaning "yellow" (see Illustration 27).

The corpus luteum then begins to make another hormone. This hormone is called *progesterone*, and it travels to the uterus and causes the endometrium to grow still thicker and to make nourishing substances that can help a fertilized ovum develop and grow into a baby.

If the ovum has been fertilized and the woman is going to have a baby, the corpus luteum keeps on making progesterone for a while, so that endometrium will continue to secrete the nourishment the baby will need. If the ovum hasn't been fertilized, the corpus luteum stops making progesterone and disintegrates within a few days. Without the help of the hormone progesterone, the lining of the uterus begins to break down. The spongy tissue and blood of the lining fall off the wall of the uterus, collect on the bottom of the uterus, and dribble through the cervical canal and out the os, into the vagina. (See Illustration 5 on page 15.) From there, the blood and tissues trickle down the vaginal walls

endometrium (en-doe-MEE-tree-um)
corpus (KOR-pus)
luteum (LOOT-ee-um)
progesterone (pro-JES-teh-roan)

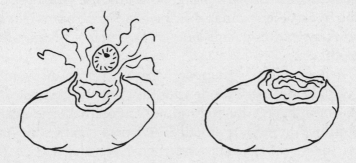

Illustration 27. Corpus Luteum. After the follicle containing the ovum has burst open, the remnants of the burst follicle turn bright yellow. These remnants are referred to as the corpus luteum.

and out the vaginal opening, and a girl has her menstrual period. The bleeding continues for a few days and then stops.

The Menstrual Cycle and Menopause

After a girl has had her first period, she continues ovulating (popping a ripe ovum off her ovary) and having her period (bleeding for a few days) about once a month for many, many years. This monthly process of ovaluating and menstruating is called the *menstrual cycle*. Although the menstrual cycle repeats itself for many years, it does not continue forever. Once a woman reaches a certain age, usually between forty-five and fifty-five, her ovaries stop producing a ripe ovum each month, and she no longer has her monthly bleeding period. Just as we have the word *puberty* for the time in a young woman's life when she first *starts* ovulating and menstruating, so we have a word for the time in an older woman's life when she *stops* ovulating and menstruating. This time in a woman's life is called *menopause*.

Menopause may happen very abruptly. A woman may have her period one month, then the next month she doesn't have her period and never has one again. Or it may happen gradually. A woman may skip one, two (or more) periods, and then have one or two (or more periods), skip some and then have her period again for a while, and so on, until she finally stops altogether.*

As a woman is going through menopause, her body is making less of the hormones estrogen and progesterone. Most women adjust to this change in their body chemistry with no problems. Some women have hot flashes, brief episodes in which their body heats up and they perspire profusely, as they are going through menopause. For most women, hot flashes, although bothersome, are not so severe that they need a doctor's care, but a few women have such severe and frequent hot flashes that they need to seek medical care to help in controlling them.

Just as there are many myths and misconceptions about hymens and about masturbation, so there are many myths about menopause. Women going through menopause, or the "change of life," as it is sometimes

menopause (MEN-o-pause)

*Menopause is not the only reason women skip menstrual periods; see pages 142–43 for more details.

called, supposedly are prone to fits of depression, anxiety, or crazy behavior. People used to think that a woman going through menopause would suddenly grow old, develop wrinkles, get fat, and feel less sexual desire. Today we know that menopause doesn't really cause any of these things. But there are many people who still have myths and misconceptions about menopause, so you may hear some of these things. If so, just ignore them.

But menopause is many years away for you, and you're probably more interested in learning about how menstruation works and about having your first period. We'll be talking about these things in the next chapter, but first we'd like to answer a question that always comes up in my class question box when we talk about the reproductive organs: "Can a person be born with both male and female sex organs?"

Hermaphrodites

The answer is yes. People who are born with both male and female sex organs are called *hermaphrodites.*

Hermaphrodites have both testicles and ovaries on the inside of their bodies. On the outside, a hermaphrodite might have a penis, a man's body build, and a beard, but have breasts like a woman. A hermaphrodite can also look like a woman, with a curvy body shape, breasts, and no beard, but have a penis instead of female genital organs, or have a vulva with inner and outer lips but a penis instead of a clitoris. There are any number of different ways that a hermaphrodite might look,

hermaphrodite (her-MAF-row-dite)

and sometimes their genital organs don't quite look like those of either sex.

Most of the time, it's obvious right from the moment of birth that a person is a hermaphrodite because of the way the genital organs look. But occasionally a hermaphrodite will have normal-looking genital organs at birth and throughout childhood, so everyone assumes the person is either male or female (depending on which kind of genital organs the hermaphrodite has). But, when puberty starts, it becomes obvious that this person is a hermaphrodite. For instance, a hermaphrodite who has normal-looking male sex organs during childhood may start to grow breasts during puberty. Or a hermaphrodite who has normal-looking female sex organs during childhood may develop a male body shape, grow a beard, and fail to start menstruating and to develop breasts.

When I explain to my class about hermaphrodites, I usually see a few kids gulping and looking very nervous and worried. The girls who haven't had their menstrual periods or whose breasts haven't begun developing start wondering if they really are females. If the other girls their age have started their periods and to develop breasts and they haven't, or if (like many girls) they've started to grow some dark hairs on their upper lips, then they start worrying, "Oh, no, maybe I'm a hermaphrodite!" Some of the boys usually look worried, too, especially if they've noticed their breasts swelling (many boys' breasts swell a bit as they are going through puberty).

I tell them not to worry. For one thing, hermaphroditism is *very, very* rare. Besides, if they were hermaphrodites, they'd already know it. It's usually obvious right from the moment a baby is born. (Nowadays, doctors are able to do special plastic surgery operations on the sex organs on the outside of the body so the child will grow up looking like a normal male or female, depending on which sex is most appropriate in that particular child's case. So, today, most hermaphrodites grow up looking quite normal, though their reproductive organs usually don't work right; they may have to take certain hormones and they usually aren't able to have children.)

But, enough of this, let's move on to the menstrual cycle and having your first period.

CHAPTER 7

The Monthly Miracle: The Menstrual Cycle

Once a month, deep inside our bodies, the ovary begins, ever so slowly, to change. The bubble on its surface contains the one ovum that has, for some mysterious reason, been chosen from all the hundreds of thousands of ova to be released that month. The funnel-like opening at the end of the fallopian tube, lined with thousands of undulating cilia, turns to meet the ovary.

Suddenly, the bubble bursts. Triggered by a spurt of luteinizing hormone, the chemical messenger from the pituitary, the ovary contracts sharply and the ripe ovum bursts forth. The fringed ends of the fallopian tubes reach out like fingers to grasp the ripe ovum and draw it into the narrow tunnel of the tube. In a dream-like, slow-motion ballet, the tiny cilia caress the ripe ovum and gently move it along on its four-inch, four-day journey to the uterus.

As the ovum is moving through the tube toward the uterus, the lining of the uterus is preparing itself. The blood vessels in the area swell, flooding the uterus with a rich supply of blood to nourish the soft, spongy tissue of the uterine lining, which will cushion the ovum when it arrives. Glands in the uterus pour forth a banquet of nutrients that will nourish the developing ovum. The lining of the uterus has thickened to twice its normal depth—a luxuriously rich topsoil in which the ovum, if fertilized during the journey through the tube, will implant.

For the first three days after its arrival, the tiny ovum floats freely within the plush uterus. If fertilized, it will embed itself in the uterus on the seventh day. Meanwhile, on the surface of the ovary, the remnant of the burst bubble, the corpus luteum, which has turned a bright yellow after its explosive spasm, awaits a message from the uterus.

If in the upper reaches of the dark, narrow fallopian tube no sperm meets and fertilizes the ovum, the ovum will not implant in the lining of the uterus. Then the corpus luteum begins to disintegrate. The chemical messages it's been transmitting to the uterus via the hormone progesterone cease. The levels of progesterone in the bloodstream drop. Without the continued supply of progesterone from the corpus luteum, the swollen network of blood vessels shrinks, restricting the flow of blood to the lining. This deprives the newly grown tissues in the lining of their support and nourishment. Over a period of days, the lining falls away in small pieces. Within hours the now weakened blood vessels of the lining open, a few at a time. Each tiny vessel empties its droplets. More and more droplets are released and the flow of menstrual blood empties the uterus of the no-longer-needed tissues.

After some days of bleeding, the lining is emptied out and this process begins all over again. The uterine lining starts to grow rich and thick again, and more ova begin to move toward the surface of the ovary. Another ovum is released at ovulation, and if the woman is not going to have a baby, then her period begins again about two weeks after ovulation.

The Menstrual Cycle

The time from the first day of bleeding of one menstrual period to the first day of bleeding of the next period— the menstrual cycle—takes about a month. The menstrual cycle may last for anywhere from twenty-one to thirty-five days. The average is about twenty-eight days. But there are very few women who actually have their periods regularly, every twenty-eight days, like clockwork, throughout their entire lives. Most of us are somewhat more irregular than this. For example, in the last year, my periods went like this: My first three periods of the year were very regular. I began to bleed once every twenty-nine days, and the bleeding lasted for five days each time. My fourth period came twenty-seven days after my third and lasted for only four days. Then I didn't have a period again for thirty days, and when I did have it, it lasted for six days. My next period came thirty-one days later and lasted for five days. Then I started having my periods more regularly again, once every twenty-nine days, and I bled for five days each time.

Each of us has her own pattern. Some are more regular than others. We may be very regular and suddenly get irregular, as one woman explained:

> I was very regular when I was younger. I could set my watch by it, once every twenty-six days. Then, when I

turned thirty, I got real irregular—once every twenty-two days, once every twenty-six, once every thirty. Now, I'm more regular again.

On the other hand, some women are very irregular and then suddenly their periods start to get regular. No one is exactly sure why some women are regular and others irregular or why our patterns may change. But we do know that traveling, emotional ups and downs, illness, and such things can affect our menstrual periods, making them start earlier or later than usual. There is an old-wives' tale that says that women who live together, who spend a lot of time with each other, or who are close friends tend to have their periods around the same time, which might also account for why our patterns change. "That's certainly true for me," one woman told us:

> I've always menstruated about the same time as the other women I'm around. When I lived at home, my sisters and I always had our periods together at the beginning of each month. When I went away to college, I found that my periods changed. I started menstruating around the middle of the month, same as my roommates.

As it turns out, this old-wives' tale may have a great deal of truth to it. Scientific studies have shown that women who are close do often have their periods around the same time.

Young women who've just started having their periods are particularly likely to have irregular periods. It takes a while for our bodies to adjust to menstruating. You may have your first period and not have another one for six months. Or you may have your second period two weeks after your first one. It often takes two or three years to develop anything near a regular pattern, and some of us never do get very regular.

Length of Your Period/Amount and Type of Blood Flow

Your period may last anywhere from two to seven days. The average is about five days. Some of your periods may last longer than others, so one month you may bleed for only two or three days, and the next time you may bleed for five or six days. Or you may be one of those women who bleeds for exactly five days each time. Here again, each of us has our own individual pattern, and our patterns may change over the course of our lives.

Although it may seem as if a lot of blood comes out of the uterus, it isn't really that much. The amount of blood may vary from one tablespoon to one cup. Women have different patterns in this too. Some of us always have heavy periods, about eight tablespoons each time; others always have light periods, only one tablespoon each time. Still others vary between having heavy and light periods.

Some of us tend to bleed most heavily on the first day or two, gradually trickling off until there is only a light flow of blood on the last day. Others start off lightly on the first day, then get heavier. Still others will bleed for a number of days and stop or slow down to only a trickle for a day or so, then bleed more heavily again. All these patterns, or any combination of these patterns, is normal.

The blood and tissue that comprise the menstrual flow may be thin and watery, or the flow may have thick clumps called clots. You may be more apt to notice clots in the morning when you get up, for the blood has been pooling and congealing in the top of the vagina while you've been lying down asleep.

The blood may be bright red to brown in color. It is

especially likely to be brownish at the very beginning or toward the end of your period. Blood tends to turn brown the longer it sits. If your blood has been slow in moving out of your body, it may take on a brownish color.

The Four Phases

Regardless of whether your periods usually come every twenty-one days or every thirty-five days, whether they're regular or irregular, light or heavy, the menstrual cycle works in essentially the same way in all of us. The menstrual cycle can be divided into four parts, or phases.

PHASE 1

The first phase of the menstrual cycle is the bleeding phase, when you are actually having your period. During this phase, the uterine lining is breaking down and being shed. We call the first day of bleeding Day 1 of your menstrual cycle. As we said, the bleeding phase may last for one to seven days, but it usually lasts about five days. So, for purposes of this discussion, we'll call Day 1 to Day 5 the first, or bleeding, phase of the cycle (see Illustration 28).

PHASE 2

During this phase, the pituitary gland is making FSH, which causes the follicles in the ovary to make estrogen and to move toward the surface of the ovary. The estrogen also causes the lining of the uterus to develop new blood passageways and spongy tissues to cushion them.

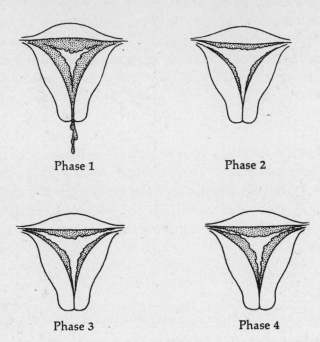

Phase 1   Phase 2

Phase 3   Phase 4

Illustration 28. The Uterus in the Four Stages of the Menstrual Cycle

In a woman with a twenty-eight-day cycle who bleeds for five days, this phase would start on about Day 6 and would continue until Day 13 or so. Of course, if your cycle is longer or shorter than twenty-eight days, this phase may be longer or shorter.

PHASE 3

By the end of Phase 2, the ovaries are making enough estrogen so that the pituitary gland slows down its production of FSH and releases a spurt of LH. The LH travels to the ovary and causes the bubble on the surface of the ovary that contains the ripe ovum to pop. This phase is, then, the ovulation phase, the phase in which the ripe egg is released from the ovary.

Generally, the ovaries only produce one ripe ovum during each menstrual cycle. Scientists believe that the ovaries take turns. During one cycle, the right ovary ovulates, and during the following cycle, the left ovary does. If a woman only has one ovary, either because she was born with only one or one has been removed because it was diseased, then the remaining ovary takes over and produces a ripe ovum each month.

Most women don't feel anything when the bubble bursts and the ripe ovum pops off the ovary; however, some women do know when they are ovulating because they feel a cramp or a pain. Some women have a dull achy feeling for a day or so around the time they are ovulating. Others have a sudden sharp pain that passes very quickly; still others experience just a mild twinge that is hardly noticeable. But for most of us ovulation happens without our being aware of it.

In a woman with a twenty-eight-day cycle, ovulation usually occurs on Day 14; however, it may happen one or two days earlier or later than this—that is, anywhere from Day 12 to Day 16.

Most books that describe the menstrual cycle talk about a twenty-eight-day cycle and explain that ovulation occurs about halfway through the cycle, on Day 14. Women who have longer or shorter cycles often assume that they too will ovulate at the halfway point of their cycles. Thus, many women think that ovulation would occur halfway through a thirty-two-day cycle, on about Day 16, or halfway in a twenty-two-day cycle, on Day 11. This is not true. Ovulation occurs about fourteen days (give or take one or two days either way) before the first day of bleeding of the next period. So, if a woman has a thirty-two-day cycle, she probably ovulates around Day 18 (32 — 14 = 18), and if she has a twenty-two-day cycle, she probably ovulates around Day 8 (22 — 14 = 8).

A woman can get pregnant only during the ovulation phase of her menstrual cycle, when her ovary has just recently released the ripe ovum. It would be nice if we could predict exactly when a woman is going to ovulate. That way, a woman who wanted to get pregnant could have sexual intercourse at a time when her chances of getting pregnant are highest, and a woman who didn't want to get pregnant could avoid having intercourse at this time. But it doesn't work that way. One month a woman might have a twenty-eight-day cycle so she'd ovulate around Day 14. But the next month she might have a thirty-five-day cycle, so she'd probably ovulate around Day 21. The following cycle might only be twenty-one days long, so she'd ovulate around Day 7.

Attempting to prevent pregnancy by trying to figure out when you are going to ovulate and avoiding sex at that time doesn't work very well. This method of preventing pregnancy, this method of birth control, is referred to as the *rhythm method*. There are other, more effective methods of birth control. If you are interested in learning more about birth control, there are a number of excellent books that talk about it (see "For Further Reading"). You might want to talk to your mother and other women to find out what, if any, method of birth control they use. If you are just starting to menstruate, you probably won't be having intercourse, so you won't need to concern yourself with birth control for a number of years. But it's a good idea to start learning about these things when you are young, so that when you do begin to have sexual intercourse, you are well informed.

PHASE 4

As this phase begins, the ripe ovum is in the fallopian tube, traveling toward the uterus. The corpus luteum, the remnants of the burst follicle on the surface of the ovary, has turned a bright yellow color and is making progesterone. The progesterone is causing the lining of the uterus to get even thicker and to secrete nutrients.

If a sperm manages to make its way into the fallopian tube at this time, there's a good chance that fertilization will take place. The sperm penetrates the outer shell of the ovum, and the fertilized ovum then travels to the uterus. It plants itself in the rich uterine lining.

If fertilization takes place, the corpus luteum continues to produce progesterone for a while so that the uterine lining will provide nutrients to nourish the fertilized ovum. But most of the time fertilization doesn't happen. The ovum disintegrates. Because fertilization hasn't happened, the corpus luteum also stops producing progesterone and it disintegrates.

At this point in the menstrual cycle there is very little estrogen and very little progesterone being made in our bodies, so the lining of the uterus starts to break down and is shed. As the lining is being shed, the pituitary starts making more FSH. In turn, the ovaries start making more estrogen. As soon as the lining is shed, a new lining begins to thicken, and the menstrual cycle starts all over again.

In a woman with a twenty-eight-day cycle, Phase 4 would run from about Day 15 (right after ovulation) until Day 28. On the twenty-ninth day, the bleeding would start again and thus would be Day 1 of the next cycle.

SUMMARY OF THE FOUR PHASES OF THE MENSTRUAL CYCLE

Phase 1
- The uterine lining is being shed; the woman is having her period.
- The pituitary and the ovaries are only making small amounts of hormones.

Phase 2
- The pituitary is making FSH.
- The ovaries are making estrogen.
- The follicles in the ovary are moving toward the surface of the ovary.
- The uterine lining is starting to thicken.

Phase 3
- The pituitary releases a spurt of LH.
- The ripe ovum bursts from the ovary and moves into the fallopian tube.

Phase 4
- The remnants of the burst follicle become the corpus luteum and begin to make progesterone.
- The progesterone makes the uterine lining grow even thicker.
- If fertilization occurs, the corpus luteum keeps making progesterone; if not, the corpus luteum disintegrates.
- Without progesterone from the corpus luteum, the uterine lining breaks down and is shed. The first day of bleeding is Day 1 of the next cycle.

Cervical Mucus Changes

In addition to the menstrual cycle changes, there are other important cyclical changes that take place in your body each month. As you may recall from the last chapter (see page 89), your cervix has certain glands which produce mucus. This mucus mixes with the old cells and cleansing fluids in your vagina to make up your vaginal discharge. The amount and type of mucus produced by these glands varies depending on the phase of the menstrual cycle.

These changes in the amount and type of your cervical mucus (and, therefore, in your vaginal discharge) may not be as noticeable in teenagers as they are in older women. The cervical mucus cycle may also follow a somewhat different pattern in different women, and for some women these changes may be more noticeable than in other women. In general, however, the pattern of cervical mucus changes goes something like this: on the days immediately following a woman's menstrual period, the glands in the cervix are not very active. They don't produce much mucus, so there is usually less vaginal discharge at this time, and the vagina and vaginal lips are apt to feel rather dry.

After a few days, the glands start to become more active, so there is an increasing amount of vaginal discharge, and the vagina and vaginal lips are noticeably "wetter." The mucus produced by the glands on these days may be clear to white to yellowish in color. It may be thin and watery or rather thick, pasty, and sticky.

During the ovulation phase of the menstrual cycle, the glands in the cervix are very active and usually produce more mucus than at any other point in the cycle. The mucus on these days tends to be clear and quite slippery. If you were to put some of this mucus between your thumb and forefinger, you would be able to stretch the mucus in long, shimmery strands. This type of mucus is called fertile mucus because it appears at the time of the month when a woman is ovulating and is therefore most fertile, or most likely to get pregnant. The mucus produced at other times of the month has a chemical makeup that is hostile to sperm and helps prevent them from passing through the cervix and into the uterus. But, this fertile mucus has a different chemical makeup that actually helps sperm on their journey and increases a woman's chances of getting pregnant.

In a few women, the fertile mucus may be accompanied by some red or brownish color in the vaginal discharge. This slight staining is not very common, but it is perfectly normal and natural, just a bit of bleeding that some women have at ovulation.

Within one to about three days after ovulation, the fertile mucus disappears. Some women don't have much mucus or discharge on these days. From this point until their next period, their vagina and vaginal lips again feel rather dry. Other women continue to have some discharge and a feeling of wetness, but the mucus on these days tends to be rather sticky and pasty, quite different from the fertile mucus. Still other women alternate between dry and wet days.

Menstruation—When?

The girls in my class always want to know, "When will I have my first period?" Unfortunately, I can't answer that question. Each of us has our own timetable. No one can say exactly when it will happen, but I *can* give you an idea. A girl may have her first period any time between her eighth and sixteenth birthdays. But very few girls have their periods when they are as young as eight, and the vast majority have theirs before they are sixteen. In fact, most girls have their periods between their eleventh and fourteenth birthdays. Still, there are plenty of girls who have their periods when they are only eight or nine and plenty who don't have theirs until fifteen or sixteen. If you reach the age of sixteen and have not started menstruating, it's a good idea to see a gynecologist, a doctor who specializes in women's health care. Not menstruating by the age of sixteen isn't necessarily a sign that there's something wrong. There have been cases of perfectly normal girls who didn't start to menstruate until their twenties, but it's a good idea to see a doctor to rule out the possibility that you have a medical problem that is keeping you from menstruating.

Even though it's impossible to say exactly when any particular girl will have her first period, there are some clues. One thing that may give you a clue as to when you'll start is when your mother started. Daughters often have their first periods around the same age that their mothers did. This is not a hard-and-fast rule, but it is at least a clue. See if your mom can remember exactly when she started.

You might want to use the chart on page 119 to keep track of your progress through puberty. Perhaps keeping a chart like this is something you and your mom, a girlfriend, or another person you feel close to could do together, and it might be fun to share this chart with your daughter if someday you become the mother of a girl.

Start by filling in the first section of the chart. Every three months or so fill in a new section. (Make more chart pages as you need them.) Begin by writing in the date and recording your height and weight. If you have not yet begun your growth spurt, you may notice a dramatic increase in your height and weight as time passes and you fill in more sections on the chart. If

gynecologist (GUY-neh-KOL-oh-jist)

your growth spurt has already started, you'll probably notice a more gradual increase in your height and weight.

On the next line, where it says "Stage of Pubic Hair Development," write the numeral 1, 2, 3, 4, or 5 to indicate which stage of pubic hair development you are in now. It might be helpful to turn back to Illustration 8, on page 27, which shows the five stages of pubic hair development. If you don't have any pubic hairs at all, you would write the numeral 1 on that line of the chart. If you have at least a few pubic hairs, you would write the numeral 2 there. If your pubic hair looks more like the drawing of Stage 3, write a 3, and so on. If you are between stages, you might want to write something like "between Stage 2 and 3" or "between Stage 3 and 4."

On the next line, the one that says "Stage of Breast Development," write the stage you are closest to right now. It might be helpful to look at Illustration 11 on page 49. Again, if you're between stages, you might want to make a note of this.

If you notice other changes, for example, underarm hair, dark hair on your arms and legs, more perspiration, pimples, a change in the appearance of your vulva, a vaginal discharge—note these things on your chart in the space after the words "Other Changes." Any time you notice something new, fill in another section of the chart, even if it hasn't been three months since your last entry. Of course, when you first menstruate, mark that on the chart too!

Keeping a chart like this of the stages of pubic hair and breast development can give you some idea of when you'll start to menstruate. Doctors have studied groups of girls going through puberty to see what

MY PUBERTY CHART

Date:
Height: Weight:
Stage of Pubic Hair
  Development:
Stage of Breast
  Development:
Other Changes:

Date:
Height: Weight:
Stage of Pubic Hair
  Development:
Stage of Breast
  Development:
Other Changes:

Date:
Height: Weight:
Stage of Pubic Hair
  Development:
Stage of Breast
  Development:
Other Changes:

Date:
Height: Weight:
Stage of Pubic Hair
  Development:
Stage of Breast
  Development:
Other Changes:

Date:
Height: Weight:
Stage of Pubic Hair
  Development:
Stage of Breast
  Development:
Other Changes:

Date:
Height: Weight:
Stage of Pubic Hair
  Development:
Stage of Breast
  Development:
Other Changes:

Date:
Height: Weight:
Stage of Pubic Hair
  Development:
Stage of Breast
  Development:
Other Changes:

Date:
Height: Weight:
Stage of Pubic Hair
  Development:
Stage of Breast
  Development:
Other Changes:

stages of breast and pubic development girls were in when they started to menstruate. The following table shows the results of these studies.

WHEN GIRLS STARTED TO MENSTRUATE

Stage	Percentage* of girls who started to menstruate in each stage of breast development	Percentage* of girls who started to menstruate in each stage of pubic hair hair growth
1	0%	0%
2	1%	4%
3	26%	19%
4	62%	63%
5	11%	14%

* Percentage means part of 100. If we say 62 percent of all girls menstruate when they are in breast Stage 4, we mean that of a group of 100 girls, 62 of them will have their first period while they are in Stage 4 of breast development.

As you can see from this table, most girls (62 percent) start to menstruate when they are in Stage 4 of breast development. Also, most girls (63 percent) have their first periods in Stage 4 of pubic hair development. So if your puberty chart shows you've reached Stage 4 of breast and pubic hair development, you can expect to start menstruating in the near future. However, as you can also see from the table, 11 percent of girls don't have their periods until Stage 5 of breast development and 14 percent don't start until Stage 5 of pubic hair development. Moreover, a fair number of girls, 26 percent, start their periods while they are in breast Stage 3, and 19 percent start while they are in pubic hair Stage 3.

None of the girls studied started to menstruate while they were in breast Stage 1 or in pubic hair Stage 1. So if you are still in Stage 1, you probably won't start menstruating until you've moved to a more advanced stage of breast and pubic hair development.

Breast development and pubic hair development don't always go together. So you may be in one stage of breast development and in another stage of pubic hair development. For example, one of the girls in my class had her first period when she was in Stage 4 of breast development and Stage 3 of pubic hair development.

Another question that often comes up in my classes is, "How long does it take to go through the various stages?" Again it's hard to answer this question exactly, but we do know how long most girls take to go through them.

LENGTH OF TIME THAT GIRLS REMAIN IN VARIOUS STAGES

Stage	Most Girls	95 Percent of All Girls
Breast Stage 2	About 11 months	About 2½ to 12 months
Breast Stage 3	About 11 months	About 4 to 26 months
Breast Stage 4	24 months	About 1 month to 7 years
Pubic Hair Stage 2	About 7 months	About 2½ to 15½ months
Pubic Hair Stage 3	6 months	About 2½ to 11 months
Pubic Hair Stage 4	About 15½ months	About 7 to 29 months

As you can see, most girls spend about eleven months in Stage 2 of breast development. In other words, it takes eleven months to get from the beginning of Stage 2 to the beginning of Stage 3. But that's only most girls. Some girls take as little as two-and-one-half months and some as long as twelve months. There are a few girls (about 5 percent) who will take either a shorter or longer time than this.

Likewise, reading across the second line of the table will tell you that most girls spend about eleven months in breast Stage 3. Some girls take as little as one month to get through Stage 3 and some take as many as twenty-six months. Ninety-five percent of us will take somewhere between one and twenty-six months; most of us will take about eleven months.

Your First Period

These charts and tables are fun to fool around with and they can give you some idea of when you can expect to start menstruating, but no one can predict the exact day of your first period and this worries many girls.

"What'll I do if it happens when I'm at school?" is a question that often comes up in my classes. Luckily, there are usually some girls in my classes who've already started to menstruate and can share their experiences with the other girls. Here's what one of them had to say:

> I got my first period during history class. I wasn't sure if it was happening, but I sort of knew. So I raised my hand and said I had to go to the bathroom. Sure enough, there was blood on my underpants. Luckily, I had my purse with some change in it, so I got a sanitary napkin out of the machine and pinned it to my underpants and just went back to class.

Sanitary napkins are pads of soft cotton that are used to absorb the menstrual flow. This girl was lucky. There was a napkin machine in the girl's room and she had some change with her. Another girl wasn't so lucky:

> I got my period at school, too. I kinda knew right away
> what it was, but I went to the bathroom to check. There
> weren't any napkins in the machine, so I just wadded up
> some toilet paper and went to the nurse's office. She was
> real nice and gave me a clean pair of underpants and a
> napkin.

A number of girls said that they'd gone to the school
nurse, to their gym teachers, to the secretary in the
school office, or to a woman teacher for a sanitary
napkin. If their underpants were bloody, sometimes the
nurse or whoever had a spare pair. At other times,
they'd just ignored the blood or they'd just rinsed their
pants out with cold water and put them on while they
were still damp or waited until they dried. Other girls
said they'd gone to a telephone and called their moms
who'd come to school with clean pants and napkins.

One girl told us that she'd been prepared:

> I knew I was getting old enough, so at the beginning of
> seventh grade, I put a sanitary napkin in my purse in
> those special carrying cases they give you. And I just
> kept it there so I'd be ready. The school I was going to
> didn't have a school nurse, and the napkin machines
> were always broken or empty. I didn't want to have to
> go into the office and say I was having my period and
> needed a napkin. There were always a lot of people in
> there. I would have been so embarrassed.

Another girl told us that she, too, had been prepared:

> I had that napkin in my purse for almost a year. I thought
> I was so smart—being ready and all.
>   Then I'm walking down the hall one day and my girl
> friend says, "Hey, you got blood on your skirt." I almost
> died. "Stand in back of me," I said, and she walked down
> the hall kind of right behind me, so no one could see. I
> got my coat out of my locker and put it on and went to
> the office. I told the secretary I was sick and had to go
> home.

Most girls notice a feeling of wetness before the blood soaks through their underpants and onto their clothes. And most girls don't bleed enough right at first to have it show through on their clothes. But some girls had embarrassing stories to tell about how the blood had soaked through their clothes, making a spot. If you're feeling worried about your first period, why not talk it over with your mom or someone else who might have some helpful hints. Finding out what has happened to other people or just talking about your worries can help a lot.

Sanitary Napkins, Tampons, and Sponges

You can have your period any time, night or day, at home, at school, or anywhere you happen to be. Regardless of where or when it happens, you'll want to have some way of absorbing the menstrual flow.

In the past, women have used everything from grass to soft cloths and sponges to catch their menstrual flow. Nowadays, we have all sorts of menstrual products, so many that it may be hard to choose which ones you want to use. You might ask your mom or another woman which she prefers and why. You can also try the various products yourself until you hit on the ones you like best.

SANITARY NAPKINS OR PADS

Sanitary napkins come in different sizes and thicknesses and can be bought in supermarkets and drugstores. They are made of layers of soft cotton. Most of them have a piece of plastic lining to prevent the blood from soaking through the pad (see Illustration 29).

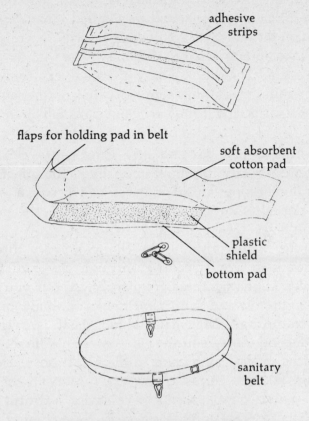

Illustration 29. Sanitary Napkins

Some sanitary napkins are made to be worn with a belt. The napkin fits to the belt, which is worn around the waist. You can also pin the napkin to your underpants with safety pins. Some napkins are made so that you don't need pins or a belt. They have a strip of sticky adhesive on the underside. The adhesive is covered by a strip of glossy paper. You remove the strip of paper and press the napkin onto your underpants. The adhesive will hold the napkin in place.

If you have a heavy menstrual flow, you may need to use the thickest pads (sometimes called "maxi" pads), at least on the days you are flowing heavily. If your flow is lighter, you may want to use one of the thinner pads, which are not as bulky. There are also very thin pads (called "mini" pads) that some girls use on the last day or so of their period if they only have a small amount of blood.

Wearing a pad for the first time can feel rather strange, especially the thick ones. Even though it may feel as if everyone can see that you're wearing a pad, it really doesn't show. Check yourself out in the mirror and you'll see—the pad really isn't visible.

Sanitary napkins should be changed every three or four hours to avoid soaking through the pad. It's a good idea to change them frequently, even if you have a very light flow and don't have to worry about soaking through the pad. Menstrual blood itself is perfectly clean and odorless, but once it comes in contact with the germs in the vagina and in the air, it does develop an odor, because germs grow very rapidly in the rich blood. These germs aren't necessarily harmful, but they can cause an unpleasant odor. By changing your pad frequently, you won't give the germs and odor a chance to develop.

Used napkins should be put in a wastebasket or trashcan. Don't flush them down the toilet, as they will clog the plumbing. Public bathrooms often have special disposal containers for sanitary napkins right in the toilet stall. If there isn't one and you don't want to come waltzing out of the stall in front of everyone with a bloody napkin in your hand, fold the napkin in half and wrap it in toilet paper. Then, when you leave the stall, just toss it in the nearest trashcan. It's a good idea to wrap them up like this even when you're at home, for it will cut down on odor from the pad.

TAMPONS

Another way of catching the menstrual flow is to use a tampon. Women have been using tampons since the dawn of time. They made small rolls of absorbent grass or cloth and put the roll inside the vagina to absorb the blood. Nowadays, we have tampons made of absorbent cotton that usually have a string attached to the end so they can be easily removed. Most tampons come in an applicator to make it easier to insert the tampon into the vagina.

The girls in my class usually have a lot of questions about tampons. First of all, they want to know if a tampon can "go up inside you." The answer is no. The tampon goes through the vaginal opening, into the vagina, but it can't get up into the uterus. The passage-way between the vagina and uterus, the cervical canal, is too small. The opening to the cervical canal, the cervical os, is no bigger around than the head of a matchstick. It's simply not possible for a tampon to get into the uterus.

The girls in my class also want to know whether a tampon can "get lost" in the vagina, usually because they've heard some story about a woman who had to go to the doctor because her tampon "got lost." A tampon can't really get lost in the vagina, but what can happen is that the string that is attached to the end of the tampon may get drawn up into the vagina, or the tampon may get so far into the vagina that the woman can't feel the string and thinks it's lost. If this should happen to you, relax—it's a simple matter to get it back out again. Just reach your fingers up inside your vagina and pull the tampon out. If it's way up inside there, you may have to squat or bear down as if you were making a bowel movement. This will push the tampon down lower so you can reach it. Most of the time, the tampon string dangles out of the vaginal opening and you just pull gently on the string to remove the tampon.

Girls also want to know whether a virgin, a person who has never had sexual intercourse, can use a tampon. The answer is yes. A girl can use a tampon regardless of her age and whether or not she's a virgin. It may be more difficult to use a tampon if you're young or if you only have small openings in your hymen. But your vaginal opening and your hymen are stretchy. If you have trouble getting the tampon in, try using your finger gently to stretch the opening. After a couple of months of gently stretching yourself a few times a week, you should be able to get the tampon in.

The girls in my class always want to know in exact detail how to get the tampon in. Since the instructions that come with most tampons are not very detailed, we always spend some time talking about how to insert a tampon.

Some women like to insert their tampons while they are standing up; others do it lying down; still others do it in a sitting position. Regardless of which position you use, it helps if you remember that the vagina doesn't go straight up and down, but angles toward the small of the back. If you don't insert the tampon at a slight angle, it's going to hit against the vaginal walls and will be much harder to insert.

Make sure, too, that you're using the right size tampon. Tampons, which can also be purchased in supermarkets and drugstores, come in three or four sizes. The small size may be called a regular or junior size and the largest is called a super. If you're just starting out, you will want the smallest, thinnest tampon as it will be easier to insert.

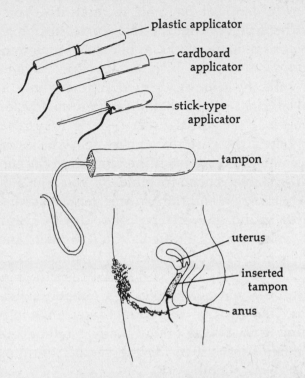

plastic applicator

cardboard
applicator

stick-type
applicator

tampon

uterus

inserted
tampon

anus

Illustration 30. Tampons

If you're using a tampon with an applicator, spend
a few minutes fooling around with one of the applica-
tors so you'll know how it works. If your vaginal opening is dry, you might want to lubricate the tampon
with a little saliva or K-Y Jelly. Don't use hand or
body lotions or face creams to lubricate the tampon;
they may contain chemicals or perfumes that could
irritate your vulva and vagina.

It's important to relax because if you are tense, your
muscles will tighten up and your vaginal opening will
contract.

Be sure to remove the outer wrapping, then gently
push the end of the tampon and applicator into your

vagina to a depth of one-half to one inch. You may have to hold one portion of the applicator while you push on the plunger of the applicator. Some tampons come on a stick. You push the tampon up into the vagina with the stick. Others don't have any applicator at all; you just push the tampon up inside with your finger.

Now here's the part they never tell you in the instructions. If you don't push the tampon in far enough, it's going to feel uncomfortable. If you put a finger inside your vagina and tighten the muscles in the area by pulling in and up, you'll feel the muscles just inside your vaginal opening tighten. You'll want to get the tampon up above the point where those muscles tighten. Otherwise, the tampon is caught between the muscles and it will feel uncomfortable. If a tampon is inserted properly, you won't be able to feel it once it's in place. And there is no danger of the tampon falling out because the muscles just inside the vaginal opening will prevent it from slipping out.

If it hurts to insert the tampon, then use a sanitary napkin and try gently stretching your opening with your finger as we explained above. Then try a tampon again.

Like napkins, tampons should be changed every three or four hours. The tampon itself can be flushed down the toilet, but the applicator should be thrown in a wastecan as it could clog the toilet.

Tampons are so comfortable to wear that women sometimes forget they're there and may neglect to remove the last one at the end of their periods. This will eventually cause a foul odor and maybe a discharge, but after you remove the forgotten tampon, this should clear up.

SPONGES

Some women use sponges to catch the menstrual flow (see Illustration 31). The advantage of the sponge is that it can be taken out and rinsed clean and reused. I have several friends who use sponges and think they're the greatest thing in the world. I've tried them, and to tell you the truth, I didn't think they were so great. They tended to "leak" blood, but what really bothered me was that it seemed impossible to rinse the blood completely out of the sponge. I don't recommend them because I'm afraid they can't be cleaned well enough to prevent infections.

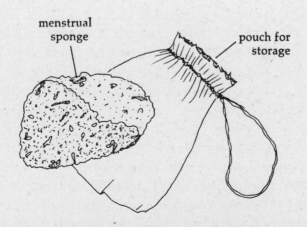

Illustration 31. Menstrual Sponge

TOXIC SHOCK SYNDROME

While we're on the subject of napkins, tampons, and sponges, we should probably mention *toxic shock syndrome* (TSS for short), which is a disease that has been associated with the use of tampons, napkins, and menstrual sponges. Most of the people who've gotten TSS have been women under the age of thirty who were having their periods at the time that they got the disease and who were using tampons or, less frequently, menstrual sponges or napkins. But males and younger and older females have also gotten TSS, as well as women who weren't menstruating at the time they came down with the disease.

TSS is an infection. When it is the result of using tampons, it starts in the vagina. It is caused by a germ that makes a poison or toxin that gets into the bloodstream. The disease usually starts with a sudden fever, vomiting, and diarrhea. Sometimes there is an accompanying headache, sore throat, or achy muscles. Within forty-eight hours, there may be a dramatic drop in blood pressure so that the person becomes very weak and groggy. A red rash that peels like sunburn may develop. The disease is rarely fatal, but a few women have died of TSS.

No one is certain what tampons have to do with the disease, but most of the women who've gotten it were using tampons at the time. The majority were using a particular brand, the RELY tampon. But some were using other brands or napkins or sponges. The disease was first widely noticed about the time that the RELY tampon came on the market. RELY contained a new, superabsorbent fiber, and proved very popular.

Some of the researchers studying TSS think that

toxic (TOK-sik)

these superabsorbent fibers are the source of the problem. One theory is that because the superabsorbent fibers can soak up so much blood, women don't change them as often. Thus, the blood stays in the vagina longer. Blood, as we mentioned, can be a breeding ground for germs. If a woman happens to have a TSS-causing germ in her vagina and the tampon is left in the vagina long enough, the germs can multiply and make enough poison so that the woman becomes ill. Other researchers feel that the roughness of these tiny superabsorbent fibers also contributes to TSS by causing microscopic scratches on the inside of the vagina. They feel that the poisons get into the bloodstream through these scratches.

When the news about TSS first came out, many women stopped using tampons. But because sanitary napkins are more bulky, can cause chafing, are more likely to have an odor, and are so much less comfortable, many women went back to tampons. TSS is a rare disease, affecting only about six in every hundred thousand women, so if you want to use tampons, you probably aren't taking a very big risk.

If you do use tampons, change your tampon every three or four hours. Always change it before you go to bed and first thing when you wake up, or better yet, use a sanitary napkin at night. If you do develop a sudden fever (over 102°) and are vomiting, remove the tampon and see your doctor right away.

Is It All Right To . . .?

The girls in my class always have questions about whether it is okay to do certain things while they're having their periods: Is it all right to take a bath or a shower? To wash my hair? To go horseback riding? To take a gym class? To have sexual intercourse? To drink cold drinks or eat cold food?

The answer to all these questions is yes. You can do anything you'd do at any other time of the month. Of course, if you're going swimming during your menstrual period, you'll want to use a tampon instead of a sanitary napkin.

You may have heard that you shouldn't shower or bathe during your period, but this simply isn't true. In fact, you are apt to perspire more heavily while you're menstruating, so a daily shower or bath may be especially important. You may have heard that cold food or drinks or strenuous exercise would cause a heavier flow, cause your period to last longer, or cause you to have cramps. Again, none of this is true. In fact, exercise can sometimes help to relieve cramps.

Douching

Douching is a way of cleansing the vagina by flushing it out. Either plain water, water and vinegar, or a commercial douche preparation can be used to flush the vagina. Some women use a syringe-type douche, which has a nozzle on one end and a bulb or container on the other end which holds the water or douche solution. The woman places the nozzle in her vagina and squeezes the bulb so water or douche solution is forced into the vagina. Some women use a bag-type douche, which has a nozzle and a tube that leads to a bag (resembling a hot water bottle), which holds the water or douche solution. When a clip is released, the water or douche solution runs through the tube and into the vagina.

douching (DOOSH-ing)

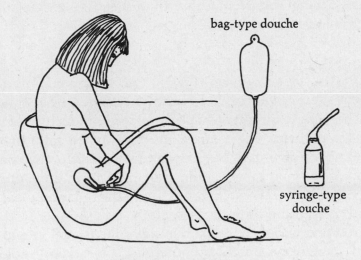

Illustration 32. Douching

Although some women do douche, it's really not a good idea. For one thing, it isn't necessary. The vagina is self-cleansing. As we've explained elsewhere, the vaginal walls secrete fluids that rinse your vagina and keep it clean naturally. These fluids are slightly acidic, which prevents germs from growing. Douching can change the acid level of your vagina and encourage infections. Commercial douche preparations can irritate your vaginal tissues. Moreover, there's always the chance of introducing germs into the vagina by means of the douche equipment. Also, excessive force could push germs from the vagina up into the uterus, causing an infection. For these reasons, it is not a good idea to douche. Occasionally, a doctor will recommend douching with certain medications as part of the treatment for a vaginal infection. Other than this, though, douching is not recommended.

Cramps

Almost every woman has cramps at some time or other in her life. They may happen before or during menstrual periods. The cramps may be just a mild achy feeling, or they may be sharp and severe. Most women only have mild cramps, and they only have them once in a while. A few women get very severe cramps each and every time they menstruate.

No one knows why women have menstrual cramps, but there are a number of theories. One theory holds that cramps happen because the uterus contracts rhythmically while we're having our periods to help expel the menstrual blood. Women who are particularly sensitive may feel these contractions as cramps. Another theory holds that cramps are caused by excessive amounts of hormones called *prostaglandins*. Prostaglandins help the uterus contract, and women who have problems with cramps often have more prostaglandins in their bodies than women who aren't troubled by cramps.

The theories go on and on. One particularly popular theory says that cramps are "all in your head." This theory is often held by doctors, who are mostly men, so maybe it's not surprising that they think "it's all in

prostaglandins (PROST-uh-glan-dins)

your head." There are plenty of women who believe this theory too, but if you've ever had severe menstrual cramps, you know it's not in your head—it's in your belly—and it hurts.

If you are troubled by cramps, exercises like the ones in Illustration 33 have proven helpful for many women.

Some women find masturbating to orgasm helpful, for after you have an orgasm, the blood vessels in the area are less congested, and blood flows more freely. Likewise, some women find that massaging their lower abdomen or using a heating pad or hot-water bottle is helpful.

If none of these remedies brings relief, you might try a pain reliever like aspirin or one of the nonaspirin pain relievers. Aspirin may be more effective than a nonaspirin pain reliever because aspirin is an anti-prostaglandin, which means it acts against the prosta-glandins. There are also aspirin-type medications, sold without prescriptions, that are made especially for menstrual pain. These medications usually contain some caffeine (the stimulant in coffee) as well. Sometimes this combination works where plain aspirin has failed.

If you've tried all these things and are still troubled by cramps, you should see a doctor. Severe cramps are sometimes a sign of some underlying medical problem. Also, a doctor can prescribe stronger pain relievers and antiprostaglandins than you can buy without a pre-scription.

If you do suffer from severe cramps, you may run into the "it's all in your head" attitude from the people around you, and from your doctor too. If so, try to ignore the people around you and find another doctor. It's very unlikely that your cramps are all in your head. Too many women have suffered too much needless

Exercise 1

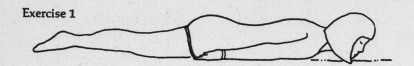

Gradually raise your head and chest without using your arms until your torso is off the floor.

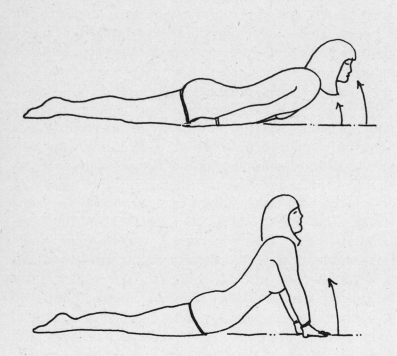

Using your arms, further raise your torso so that your back is arched. Repeat several times.

Illustration 33. Exercises for Menstrual Cramps

Exercise 2

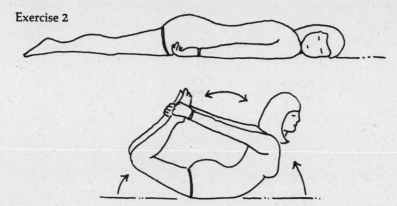

Begin by lying on your stomach. Grab your ankles with both hands, pulling forward toward the back of your head. Gently rock back and forth. Repeat several times.

Exercise 3

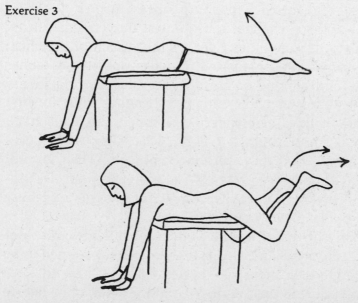

Lie on a coffee table or platform about 2–3 feet off the ground as shown here. Place your hands on the ground in front of you. Bend your knees and pull your ankles in toward your buttocks. Then in one smooth continuous motion, kick your legs out again. Continue until you gradually build up to do it for six minutes.

pain because of this "all in your head" business. If you have menstrual cramps, you deserve proper medical attention for your problem, so don't be afraid to insist upon it.

Menstrual Changes

Many women notice changes in their bodies or in their emotions that seem to take place during a certain phase of their menstrual cycle. For example, I get very energetic during my period and often get into fits of house-cleaning (which is nice because, most of the time, I'm not too enthusiastic about housework). About a week and a half before my period starts, my breasts swell a bit and get very tender, or at times downright painful. (This only started happening since I turned thirty.) I often notice a change in my bowel movements during my period. Sometimes I get a slight touch of diarrhea; other times I'm constipated for a day or so. I sometimes have mild cramps or a full, pressured feeling in my lower abdomen while I'm menstruating. On the first couple of days of my period, I sometimes get what I call the "lead vagina" feeling. My vagina and vulva feel heavy, as if they were made of lead. (Well, it's not that bad, but "lead vagina" is a pretty good description.) I always know when I'm about to ovulate because I get to feeling very sexual.

Many of the girls and women we talked to also noticed emotional and physical changes that seemed to be related to their menstrual cycles. Most of these changes happen during their periods or in the week or so before their periods. These are some of the changes you may experience while you are menstruating or just before your period starts.

extra energy
lack of energy or a tired, dragged-out feeling
sudden shifts in moods
tension or anxiety
depression
feelings of wellbeing
bursts of creativity
a craving for sweets
pimples, acne, or other skin problems
a particularly clear and rosy glow to the skin
heightened sexual feelings
headaches
vision disturbances
diarrhea
constipation
swelling of the ankles, wrists, hands, or feet
swelling and tenderness of the breasts
swelling of the abdomen
bloated feeling
temporary weight gain (usually three to five pounds)
decreased ability to concentrate
increased ability to concentrate
increased appetite
increased thirst
cramps
increased need to urinate
urinary infections
a change in vaginal discharge
nausea
runny nose
sores in the mouth
backache

In some women, these changes are very noticeable; in others, they are hardly noticeable at all; and some women don't notice any changes in their bodies or their feelings over the course of their menstrual cycles.

Premenstrual Syndrome

Some women regularly experience one or two or more of the negative menstrual changes listed above during the seven to ten days preceding their menstrual period.

Such women are said to have premenstrual syndrome, or PMS. No one is sure what causes PMS. Some doctors think PMS is related to vitamin and nutritional deficiencies; others think that PMS is caused by a hormone imbalance.

Mild forms of PMS are quite widespread. As many as 40 percent of us experience some PMS symptoms at some time in our lives. It is not unusual, for example, for a woman to have a bloated feeling, pimples, swelling of the breasts, or other PMS symptoms in the week or so before her period.

If you have mild PMS symptoms, you may find that eliminating sugar, coffee, and chocolate from your diet, eating balanced meals with foods rich in vitamin B$_6$ and magnesium (green vegetables, whole grains, nuts, and seeds), and taking a vitamin supplement that includes the B complex vitamins will help alleviate symptoms. Some doctors use hormones to treat PMS, but others are not convinced that hormone treatments are really effective.

If you think you have PMS, you should consult a doctor familiar with PMS.

Missing a Menstrual Period

If a woman gets pregnant, she stops having her menstrual period for the nine months that she is pregnant. She may start having her period again within a month or so after the baby is born, or it may take several months before she starts menstruating again. Women also miss periods as they are going through menopause. But menopause, pregnancy, and childbirth are not the only reasons why a woman sometimes misses periods. As we explained earlier, young women who've just started menstruating sometimes skip one or more periods on a regular basis. Even after a woman has been menstruating regularly for a number of years, she may occasionally skip one or more menstrual periods. This is quite normal and isn't anything to worry about; however, if you haven't had sexual intercourse with anyone and you miss three periods in a row, it's a good idea to see a doctor. Missing three periods in a row doesn't necessarily mean that there is something wrong with you. Not all women have menstrual periods every twenty-one to thirty-five days. Some women only have their periods once or twice a year; that's just the way their bodies work. But sometimes missing your periods is a sign that something is wrong. So, if you've missed three in a row, it's a good idea to see your doctor to determine whether you may have a medical problem that needs attention. If you have had sexual intercourse and you miss a period, see your doctor *right away*, for you may be pregnant.

Other Menstrual Irregularities

There are also other menstrual irregularities that happen from time to time. As we explained earlier, some months your period may be heavier than others. This is quite normal, but sometimes the bleeding is excessive. If you are soaking through a pad or tampon (and we mean literally soaking through, so it's drenched with blood) every hour for an entire day, then it's a good idea to see your doctor.

Sometimes a woman's period doesn't stop. If your period continues for more than a week without showing any signs of slowing down or letting up, once again, you should see your doctor. If you've been having your period for seven days and you're still trickling out a bit of blood, that's nothing to worry about, but if the blood is still coming out as heavily as it was in the beginning of the week, you may have a problem.

Sometimes a woman's periods come too close together. As we explained earlier, traveling, illness, emotional ups and downs can all make your period come earlier or later than usual. But if three menstrual cycles go by where your cycle is less than eighteen days or more than thirty-five days apart, it's a good idea to see your doctor.

Some women experience what we call *spotting* between their periods. Spotting is a day or two of very light bleeding. It's not unusual for a woman to spot for a day or two around the time of ovulation. You can figure out whether your bleeding is related to ovulation by keeping track of your menstrual periods (see below) and noting the days when spotting occurs. Count back two weeks from the first day of bleeding of the next cycle. If the spotting occurs around two weeks before each period, it's probably related to ovulation and isn't anything to worry about. If the spotting occurs at other times and continues for more than three cycles, again, consult your doctor.

These are just guidelines to help you decide when to see your doctor about menstrual irregularities. If you feel there's something abnormal about your periods or if you are uncertain, don't hesitate to give your doctor a call and explain the problem. The two of you can then decide whether you need an office visit. Most menstrual irregularities are not serious, but sometimes they can indicate an underlying problem that needs attention, so don't hesitate to get any problems that are bothering you checked out.

Keeping Track of Your Menstrual Cycle

It's a good idea to keep a record of your menstrual cycles. That way, you'll learn how your own pattern works and will know about when to expect your next period. (Remember, though, that you may not be very regular at first.)

You'll need a calendar. On the first day of your period, that is, on the first day of bleeding, mark an *x* on your calendar. Continue to mark an *x* for as long as the bleeding continues. When your next period starts, mark an *x* again. You might want to count the number of days between your periods and note that figure so you'll begin to get an idea of how long your menstrual cycle usually lasts (see Illustration 34).

You might also want to make a note of cramps, ovulation pain, or any of the other menstrual changes you may notice. If, for instance, you find that you have a craving for sweets, that you feel tense and cranky, or that your breasts are tender, note this on your calendar, so that you can begin to learn about your body's patterns.

S	M	T	W	Th	F	S
		1	2	3	4	5
6	7	8	~~9~~	~~10~~	~~11~~	~~12~~
~~13~~	~~14~~	15	16	17	18	19
20	21	22	23	24	25	26
27	28	29	30			

S	M	T	W	Th	F	S
				1	2	3
4	5	6	7	~~8~~	~~9~~	~~10~~
~~11~~	~~12~~	13	14	15	16	17
18	19	20	21	22	23	24
25	26	27	28	29	30	

Illustration 34. Recording Your Periods. To keep track of your periods, use a calendar like this. This girl had her first day of bleeding on the ninth and she continued to bleed for five more days, so she marked these days with *x*'s. The next cycle began on the eighth of the following month and her period lasted 5 days, which are marked with *x*'s. By counting the number of days between *x*'s, you can determine the length of your menstrual cycle. This girl's cycle was 29 days long.

CHAPTER 8

Puberty in Boys

This book was written for girls, to help them understand how puberty happens in their bodies. But puberty doesn't just happen to girls; it happens to boys, too. Since most girls are curious about boys' bodies, we decided to include a brief chapter on how puberty happens in boys (see Illustration 35).

In some ways, puberty in boys is similar to puberty in girls. In both sexes, there is a sudden growth spurt and a change in the general shape of the body. Both boys and girls begin to grow pubic hair and other body hair. Girls produce ripe ova for the first time, and boys begin to make sperm, the male counterpart of ova. The genital organs of both sexes begin to develop and grow larger. Both boys and girls begin to perspire more and tend to get pimples at this time in their lives.

But boys and girls are different, so puberty is a bit different in boys than it is in girls. For one thing,

147

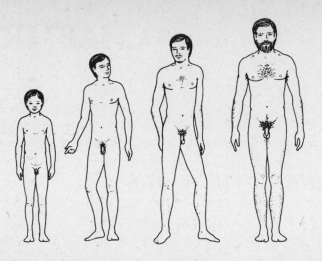

Illustration 35. Boys in Puberty. Like girls, boys too go through puberty. They get taller, their shoulders get wider, their bodies more muscular, their genital organs develop, and they begin to grow hair on their chests, arms, legs genitals, underarms, and faces.

it often *looks* as if puberty happens earlier in girls. It looks this way because, for girls, the growth spurt happens at the beginning of puberty, while for boys, it comes later in puberty. The average girl starts to develop breasts about the same time that the average boy's penis and testicles start to develop. But, with clothes on, a boy's development isn't as noticeable to others as a girl's breast development. Still, as we have seen, not everyone is average. Some girls start earlier than average, some later. The same is true of boys; some boys will actually start puberty before some of the girls their age.

Because boys and girls are different, some of the things that happen in a girl's body during puberty don't happen to boys and vice versa. Obviously, boys don't start having menstrual periods. And other things that happen to boys, such as a deepening and a lowering of the voice, don't happen to girls.

Circumcision

Illustration 1 on page 5 shows the sex organs on the outside of a man's body. You might want to take another look at that picture before reading this chapter so that you'll remember the names of the various parts of the male genitals.

Illustration 1 shows a penis that has been *circumcised. Circumcision* is an operation in which the foreskin, a sheath of skin that covers the glans, is cut away. Circumcision is usually done shortly after a boy is born, but it may also be done when a boy is older. Not all males are circumcised. If a boy or man has not been circumcised, the foreskin covers the glans. As you can see in Illustration 36, the foreskin is loose and can be stretched out or slid down the shaft of the penis so that the glans is exposed.

circumcision (sir-come-SISH-un)
circumcised (sir-come-SIZED)

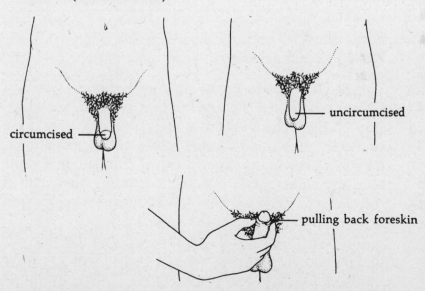

circumcised

uncircumcised

pulling back foreskin

Illustration 36. Circumcised and Uncircumcised Penis

Sometimes, a boy is circumcised for religious reasons. Some Jewish and Moslem parents have their boy babies circumcised because it was thought that men who weren't circumcised were more likely to get infections or cancer of the penis than men who had been circumcised. Doctors no longer believe that being circumcised really has anything to do with how likely it is that a man will get cancer of the penis. Besides, cancer of the penis is a rare disease. And, as long as a male washes under his foreskin regularly, he won't get infections. So, nowadays, a lot of parents are wondering whether it's really worthwhile to put a newborn baby through the pain of circumcision. More and more parents are deciding not to have their male babies circumcised.

The only difference between circumcised and uncircumcised males is that circumcised males don't have a foreskin; otherwise, their penises look, feel, and work the same way.

The Penis and Scrotum

The penis is made up of spongy tissue. There is a hollow tube called the *urethra* that runs down the inside of the penis. When a male urinates, the urine passes through this tube and comes out the opening at the tip of the glans. Sperm travel through this same tube and come out at this same opening when a man ejaculates (a valve on the bladder prevents sperm and urine from coming out at the same time).

Underneath the penis lies the scrotum, the skin sac that holds the two testicles. The testicles are very sensitive and it can be very painful if they are hit or knocked about.

Five Stages of Genital Development

The appearance of a boy's penis and scrotum changes as he goes through puberty. During childhood, a boy's scrotum is drawn up close to his body. As he goes through puberty, the scrotum begins to get looser and to hang down. When a man or boy is cold or frightened or feeling sexual, his scrotum may get tighter and draw up close to his body for a while. The penis and scrotum also get larger as a boy goes through puberty and pubic hair begins to grow around the genitals.

Just as doctors have divided the breast and pubic hair development of girls into five separate stages, so they have divided the growth of male genital organs into five stages (see Illustration 37).

Stage 1 starts at birth and continues until the boy starts Stage 2. The penis, scrotum, and testicles don't change very much during this stage, but there is a slight increase in overall size.

In Stage 2, the testicles start to grow and to hang down more. One testis may hang lower than the other. The skin of the scrotum darkens in color and gets rougher in texture. The penis gets somewhat larger.

During Stage 3, the penis gets longer and somewhat wider. The testes and scrotum continue to get larger, and the skin of the penis and scrotum may continue to get darker.

By Stage 4, the penis has gotten considerably longer and wider. The testes and scrotum have also gotten larger, and the skin of the penis and scrotum may still be getting darker.

Stage 5 is the adult stage in which the penis has reached its full width and length, and the testicles and scrotum are fully developed.

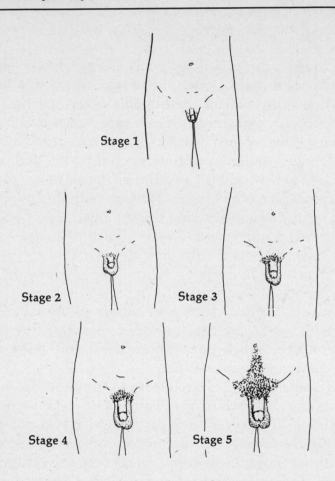

Illustration 37. The Five Stages of Male Genital Development

A boy's genitals may start developing when he is as young as nine years of age, but some boys don't start until they are fifteen or older. The average boy starts puberty after his eleventh or twelfth birthday. But, of course, not all boys are average, so some start earlier and others later. Most boys take about three or four years to go from Stage 2 to Stage 5, but some boys take less than two years, and others take five or more years.

Starting early or starting late doesn't have any effect on how long it takes a boy to go through these stages. Some early starters develop quickly, others grow slowly. The same is true for late starters: Some grow quickly, others slowly. Starting early or starting late doesn't have anything to do with how large a boy's penis will be when he's fully grown. Late starters may end up with either large or small penises, and the same goes for early starters. Just as breast size doesn't have anything to do with how feminine or womanly a female is, so penis size doesn't have anything to do with how masculine a male is.

Pubic Hair and Other Body Hair

Boys also start to grow pubic hair as they go through puberty. Boy's pubic hair is similar to girl's pubic hair. At first, there are only a few, slightly curly hairs, but as puberty continues, the hairs get curlier and darker in color, and there are more of them. The pubic hair first starts to grow around the base of the penis. Then, a few hairs begin to grow on the scrotum. As a boy gets older, pubic hair starts to grow on his lower belly and up toward his belly button. It may also grow down around his anus. It may start growing out onto his thighs. The pubic hairs usually don't start to grow until after the testes have started developing.

Boys also start to grow hair in their armpits during puberty. This usually happens about a year or so after the pubic hair has started growing, but some boys start growing hair under their arms before they have any pubic hair.

During puberty, boys also grow hair on their faces. The hair usually starts growing on the corners of the upper lips. Sideburns may start to grow at the same time. The moustache continues to grow, and then hair grows on the upper part of the cheek and just below the middle of the lower lip. Finally, it grows on the chin. Hair doesn't usually start growing on the chin until a boy's genitals are fully developed. For most boys, facial hair starts growing between the ages of fourteen and eighteen, but it may start earlier or later.

The hair on a boy's arms and legs tends to get darker and thicker during puberty. Some boys grow hair on their chests and back too. Some develop quite a bit of hair on their chests; others have very little.

Changing Shape and Size

Girls' bodies get curvier during puberty and boys' bodies get more muscular. Their shoulders get broader and their arms and legs get thicker. Boys also have a growth spurt during puberty. Their growth spurt is more dramatic than girls'. It lasts longer, and boys grow taller than girls on average. It usually happens about two years later than girls' growth spurt. Generally, it doesn't happen until their penises have started to grow.

Skin Changes

Like girls', boys' skin also begins to change during puberty. The oil glands become more active, and most boys develop some pimples. Boys, too, begin to perspire more heavily during puberty and their perspiration may have a different odor. Like girls, some boys develop purplish marks on the skin that usually appear on the hips and buttocks. As they grow older, these marks fade.

Breasts

Boys' breasts don't, of course, go through the same kind of changes that girls' do during puberty, but a boy's areola does get wider during puberty. Most boys' breasts swell a bit during puberty and, like girls, boys sometimes notice a feeling of tenderness or soreness in their breasts at this time. This swelling usually starts during Stage 2 or 3. It may happen to both breasts or only to one. It may only last a few months or a year, but it may continue for two years or even longer. Eventually, though, it goes away.

Voice

Boys' voices change during puberty, getting lower and deeper. While their voices are changing, some boys' voices have a tendency to "crack," to shift suddenly from a low pitch to a high, squeaky pitch. This cracking may only last for a few months, but sometimes it goes on for a year or two.

Erections

Way back in Chapter 1, on page 9, we talked about erections. When a man or a boy has an erection, blood rushes to the penis and fills up the spongy tissues inside the penis. Muscles at the base of the penis tighten up so the blood stays in the penis for a while, making it feel hard. During an erection, the penis gets longer and wider and, usually, darker in color, and it stands erect, away from the body as in Illustration 38.

Males get erections throughout their lives, even when they are tiny babies. Stroking or touching the penis or scrotum can cause an erection. Getting sexually excited and having sexual fantasies can cause an erection. Males can also get erections even if the penis and scrotum aren't being touched or rubbed and even if they aren't feeling or thinking about anything sexual. Some males wake up in the morning with erections. Having to urinate will cause erections sometimes.

During puberty, boys are apt to get erections more frequently. As they go through puberty, most boys start to experience what we call "spontaneous erections." Spontaneous erections are erections that happen all by themselves, without the penis or scrotum being touched or rubbed.

Spontaneous erections can be very embarrassing for a boy. They may happen when he is in school, at home, walking down the street, or just about any time or place. It's a popular myth in our society that girls are much more embarrassed by the changes that happen in their bodies during puberty—growing breasts, having their periods, and so on—than boys. But the boys in

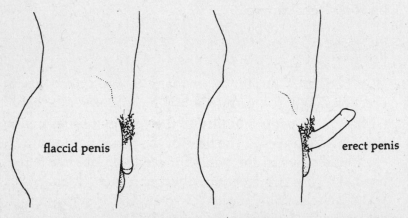

flaccid penis   erect penis

Illustration 38. Flaccid and Erect Penis. When a man or boy has an erection the soft, spongy tissue inside the penis fills with blood. The penis gets stiff and hard and stands out from his body.

my classes had a lot of stories to tell about getting spontaneous erections and worrying that the people around them would notice the bulge in their pants from the erection.

When a male has an erection, one of two things may happen. The erection may go away all by itself. The muscles at the base of the penis may relax, allowing the blood to leave the penis, so that it gets smaller and soft again. Or he may masturbate or have sexual intercourse until he has an orgasm. During an orgasm, the muscles of the penis release and contract rhythmically, and shortly after the orgasm, the muscles at the base of the penis relax, allowing the blood to leave and the penis to get soft again.

Sperm and Ejaculation

Like girls, boys begin to make their first ripe seeds, the sperm, during puberty. The cross section in Illustration 39 shows the inside of the penis and scrotum. The sperm are made inside tiny little tubes that are coiled

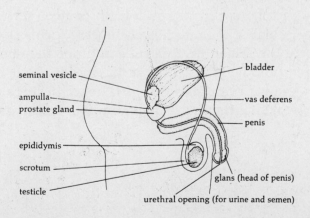

seminal vesicle
ampulla
prostate gland
epididymis
scrotum
testicle
bladder
vas deferens
penis
glans (head of penis)
urethral opening (for urine and semen)

Illustration 39. Cross Section of the Penis, Scrotum, and Testicle

up inside the testicle. They then travel through these tubes to the *epididymis*, which is a sort of storage area or compartment. The sperm spend about six weeks in the epididymis where they finish ripening. They travel from the epididymis through a tube called the *vas deferens* to another set of storage compartments located outside the testicle. These storage compartments are called the *ampulla*. Just at the lower part of the ampulla, the *seminal vesicles* connect up to the vas deferens. A fluid called seminal fluid is made in the seminal vesicles. Seminal fluid and sperm mixed together make the *semen*. The seminal fluid enriches the sperm, enabling them to swim faster. The *prostate gland* also adds some fluid to the mixture.

When a male ejaculates, the muscles of the vas deferens and prostate gland contract to force the semen out through the urethra, the tube in the center of the penis. Urine from the bladder also travels down this tube, but urine and semen can't travel through the urethra at the same time. There is a little valve on the bladder that closes off the bladder any time the semen is about to come out.

As we explained in Chapter 1, on pages 9–10, when a man ejaculates, the muscles of the erect penis contract and force the semen up this tube and out the opening in the end of the penis. Just as having her first menstrual period is a landmark for girls going through pubberty, so having the first ejaculation is a landmark for boys.

epididymis (eh-pih-DIH-dih-miss)
vas (VAS) *deferens* (DEF-eh-renz)
ampulla (am-PUL-la)
prostate (PROS-tate)
seminal (SEM-in-ul) *vesicles* (VES-eh-kuls)

A boy may have his first ejaculation while he is masturbating. Many of the boys in our class had their first ejaculations in this way. Others have their first ejaculation in their sleep. This is known as having a wet dream. The boy wakes up and finds one or two table-spoonfuls of creamy, white liquid on his belly or his bedclothes. If he hasn't been prepared for it, having a wet dream can come as quite a surprise.

Wet dreams are the male body's way of relieving the testicles of a buildup of sperm. If a boy masturbates a lot during the day, then he may not have wet dreams at night, for masturbating until he ejaculates will also empty out the buildup of sperm in the testicles.

As you can see, boys, as well as girls, go through puberty. Their bodies change and they too are getting ready for the time in their lives when they may decide to have babies.

CHAPTER 9

Sexual Intercourse, Pregnancy and Childbirth, and Birth Control

The changes that take place in boys' and girls' bodies during puberty happen because their bodies are getting ready for a time in their lives when they may want to reproduce—that is, make a baby. Many of the kids in my classes have matured to the point where they're making sperm or ovulating and are physically capable of reproduction. But they aren't ready to become parents yet, not by a long shot! In fact, if you're like most of the boys and girls in my classes, you probably spend about as much time thinking about having babies as you do thinking how you could help out around the house by doing more chores or what you'd pack to take on a trip to the moon.

reproduce (REE-preh-DOOSE)
reproduction (REE-preh-DUCK-shun)

Even though the kids in my class aren't planning to have babies any time soon, they're still curious about how babies are made, so we spend a fair amount of time in class talking about reproduction and things like sexual intercourse, pregnancy, and childbirth. I even show a videotape which shows a baby being born, and although the kids always say it's the "most totally gross thing ever," I notice that they keep begging me to show this tape year after year.

Once we've talked about intercourse, pregnancy, and childbirth in class, the kids' questions usually lead us around to another topic—ways of preventing pregnancy. So we also spend a fair amount of time talking about birth control, especially in my classes for older kids. In this chapter, we're going to be talking about these topics in pretty much the same order as we talk about them in class.

My students have about ten zillion questions on these topics. There simply isn't room in just this one chapter to answer all of them, but we'll try to answer the most commonly asked ones, and hopefully, you'll find answers to some of your questions here. If you find that some sections of this chapter are too complicated or simply don't interest you, ask for help from your parent, or skip it altogether.

Sexual Intercourse

The boys and girls in my classes and the kids who write to us are *very* curious about this topic. We explained a bit about sexual intercourse way back in Chapter 1, on pages 9–13. You may want to take another look at those pages before you read the questions and answers in this section.

I don't quite understand how the penis fits into the vagina when a man and woman have sex. Could you explain or show us a picture?
There's an old saying, "A picture is worth a thousand words," and we agree. So, we've included Illustration 40 here, which shows an erect penis fitting into the vagina in just one of the many positions a couple may use for intercourse.

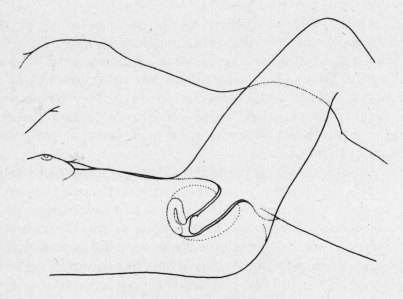

Illustration 40. Penis in vagina

What's the first thing you should do when you have sex? Could you explain to us, step by step, what people do when they're having sex?
Sexual intercourse isn't something that has specific rules you have to follow. When children go out to the play-ground after school, they don't have a specific set of directions. No one tells them that first they must take five steps, then do three somersaults, then swing on

the swing for five minutes, then climb to the top of the monkey bars. They just go out there and fool around and play and do whatever they feel like doing.

By saying this, we don't mean to suggest that having sexual intercourse is like going out to the playground to fool around (although there is a certain playfulness that can happen when two people are having sex). The point is that there just aren't any specific rules or instructions, or one "right way," to have sexual intercourse.

Some people like to hug and kiss a lot first. Touching, kissing, and hugging usually give people warm, excited, sexual feelings. The couple may then touch, rub, or caress each other's genitals or breasts before intercourse, which is called *foreplay*. They may also engage in oral-genital sex. *Oral-genital sex*, which is also called oral sex, or in slang terms "69-ing" or "a blow job," involves people using their mouths to stimulate each other's genital organs.

When questions about oral-genital sex come up in the class question box and I explain what it is, many kids go, "Oh, yuck, why would anyone want to do that?" I explain that many couples find this a very pleasurable way of enjoying each other's bodies and a special way of being close. It's also a way of being sexual with someone that doesn't involve the possibility of the woman's getting pregnant. Many kids find the idea of oral-genital sex kind of revolting because they think of this area of the body as being "dirty" or full of germs. Actually, though, this area of our bodies isn't any dirtier or more germ-laden than other parts of our bodies. In fact, most people's mouths have more germs than their genitals.

Another thing that bothers some young people when they hear about something like oral-genital sex is that they think that it's something you *have* to do when you have sex. This isn't true. Some couples enjoy oral-genital sex and often include it in their lovemaking. Others have religious or moral objections to it, or don't feel comfortable with it, so they don't do it. It's normal if you do and normal if you don't. Like everything else about sex, you're the one who decides what you do or don't want to do, and you never have to do anything that doesn't seem right for you.

Is sex painful for women?
No, sex isn't painful for women, or for men either. In fact, sex usually feels quite wonderful, provided of course that the two partners feel good about what they are doing, care about each other, and are considerate of each other's feelings.

As we've explained, the penis gets thicker and wider when it's erect, but the vagina is a very stretchy and elastic organ and easily expands to accommodate an erect penis. When a male is sexually aroused ("turned on"), his penis produces a small amount of lubricating fluid. When a female is sexually aroused, her vagina also produces lubricating fluid. These fluids help the penis slide into the vagina comfortably. In addition, the upper portion of the vagina also "balloons out" or expands somewhat when a female becomes sexually aroused, so there's usually no discomfort when the penis goes into the vagina.

If, however, a couple tries to have sex before the female is fully aroused and her vagina has begun to lubricate and expand, having sex could be uncomfortable. Since males sometimes become aroused more quickly than females, it's important for the couple to make sure that the female has enough foreplay so she is ready and well-lubricated before the penis enters the vagina.

Although sex isn't usually painful, when a female has sex for the first time (or for the first several times), she sometimes experiences some discomfort or pain. This may happen for any of a number of reasons. For one thing, she may be nervous, which makes her tighten her vaginal muscles and decreases the lubrication in her vagina. Or both partners may be rushing things, trying to put the penis into the vagina before she's lubricated enough. If the female is a virgin (a person who's never had sex before), her vaginal opening or the opening in her hymen may be rather small and tight. If the couple doesn't go slowly and gently, the hymen or vaginal opening can be painfully stretched or torn. This is why it is important for a couple to begin their sex lives in a relaxed and gentle manner.

How does it feel to have sex?
I get asked this question a lot and to tell you the truth, it's hard to answer. Sex feels different to different people. But, most people agree that it feels wonderful.

Of course, how it feels depends a lot on the situation. If you're having sex with someone you love and the two of you both feel comfortable about what you're doing, then sex can bring pleasure, fun, passion, and joy. There's a rush of good feeling when you share a good sexual experience with someone you truly care about. Sex can be a very special way of being close to someone and of discovering more about each other.

But sex can also bring sadness and emotional pain. If you don't truly care about each other or you don't feel it's right for you to be having sex, intercourse may not be a pleasant feeling at all. If you're wondering about how you'd know if it was right for you, you might read the section entitled "Making Decisions About How to Handle Your Romantic and Sexual Feelings" in the last chapter.

Pregnancy and Childbirth

Questions about pregnancy and childbirth often come up in class. Here are some of the questions that have been asked.

Are there only certain times of the month when a girl can get pregnant, and if so, when?

Yes, the ovum can be fertilized only during the thirty-six or so hours (some experts say forty-eight hours) right after it has left the ovary, because only then is it at the exact ripeness to allow for fertilization. After that, the egg is "overripe" and cannot be fertilized. Within a few days, it will break down and disintegrate completely.

Because there's only, at most, forty-eight hours during which an ovum can be fertilized in each menstrual cycle, it would seem to be a pretty easy thing to avoid getting pregnant: just don't have sex during those forty-eight hours. Unfortunately, it's not that simple. First of all, sperm can stay alive in the female's body for up to three (some experts say five) days. So, let's say a woman ovulated on the 10th day of the month. If she'd had sex on the 7th and the man had ejaculated, the sperm could still be in her body, alive and well, waiting for the ovum when it popped off the ovary on the 10th.

Also, there's no way to predict ahead of time exactly when a female is going to ovulate. A female usually ovulates twelve to sixteen days before the first day of bleeding of her next menstrual period. So we can count backwards and get an idea of when she ovulated in the previous cycle. But we *can't* tell when she'll ovulate in the next cycle because, as we've explained, menstrual cycles aren't always regular. One month, the cycle may last twenty-eight days, the next month thirty-two, and the next twenty-one. Even females who have fairly regular periods, say every twenty-seven or twenty-eight days, will occasionally have cycles that are longer or shorter than usual. So, even though there is only a short time during each month when a female can get pregnant, it's impossible to tell exactly when that time will come.

I heard that if you only have sex during your period, you won't get pregnant. Is this true?

No, females can and do become pregnant from having sex while they're having their menstrual period. A female whose period lasts for longer than seven days is more likely to get pregnant from having sex during her period. But, even a female whose period lasts seven days or less could get pregnant from having sex during this time.

Here's an example of how this might work. Say Mary starts her period on June 3rd. She bleeds for seven days, until June 9th. She has sex on June 8th, while she's still bleeding. Her next period starts on June 24th. Altogether, twenty-one days have elapsed between the first day of bleeding of her period on June 3rd and the first day of bleeding of her next period on June 24th. By counting back twelve to sixteen days from June 24th, we can figure that she probably ovulated between June 8th and June 12th. Mary was still bleeding on the 8th; she may have ovulated on the 8th; she had sex on the 8th. So, there is a chance she could get pregnant, even though she was having her period.

Even if Mary didn't ovulate until the 9th or 10th, she still might get pregnant because sperm can stay alive for at least three days. And if the experts who say that sperm can stay alive for five days are right, she might have gotten pregnant from having sex on the 8th, even if she didn't ovulate until the 12th.

Let's look at another example. Susan begins her period on August 1st. She bleeds for seven days, until August 7th. She has sex on August 7th, while she's still bleeding. Her next period starts on August 28th, which means she had a twenty-seven-day cycle. So she may have ovulated as early as August 12th. Even though she stopped bleeding on the 7th, there might still be some live sperm in her body from the time she had sex on the 7th. Therefore, if Susan ovulated on August 12th, she could have become pregnant from having had sex on the 7th while she was still menstruating.

So it is possible for a female to get pregnant from having sex during her menstrual period.

How old does a girl have to be before she can get pregnant? Could a girl ever get pregnant before she's had her first period?
Once a girl begins to ovulate and menstruate, she is physically capable of becoming pregnant. It would be next to impossible for a girl to get pregnant before she's had her first period. The only way this could occur would be if a girl happened to have sexual intercourse around the time that her ovary was getting ready to release its very first ripe ovum. The ovum could be fertilized by a sperm, and instead of having her first period two weeks later, as she normally would have, the girl could become pregnant.

But even if a girl did have sex right around the time of her first ovulation, it is still highly unlikely she would get pregnant because a girl's first ovum is really a sort of "practice" ovum. Usually it isn't fully mature, so it probably couldn't be fertilized. Thus, although it's possible, it's *highly unlikely* that a girl could get pregnant before having her first period.

Can a girl get pregnant the first time she has sex?

Yes, girls can and do get pregnant, even if they've only had sex one time.

Does a girl have to have sexual intercourse to get pregnant?

Generally speaking, the answer is yes. But even if the male didn't actually put his penis in her vagina, it would be possible for her to become pregnant if the sperm were ejaculated *near* the opening of the vagina. The sperm could swim into the vagina, up into the uterus, and into the fallopian tube, where it could fertilize the ovum. Also, even if a male were to pull his penis out of the vagina and ejaculate in such a way that none of the sperm got into the vagina or near the vaginal opening, pregnancy might still occur. As a male gets sexually aroused and his penis gets erect, a few drops of seminal fluid often appear at the tip of his penis. This fluid may contain sperm, and these sperm could cause pregnancy.

We should mention that, no matter what you've heard, a female *can't* get pregnant from kissing, masturbating herself, swimming in a pool, sitting on someone's lap, or sitting on a toilet seat. In fact, with the exception of special medical procedures that doctors use to help women who are having problems getting pregnant, there are no ways in which a female can become pregnant other than the ones we've mentioned here.

Are there some people who aren't able to have babies?

Yes. Some men and women are *infertile* or *sterile*, which means they aren't able to reproduce. A number of things

infertile (in-FER-tull)
sterile (STEH-rull)

can cause infertility. In females, infertility is often the result of scar tissue from past infections of the reproductive organs (see the section on pelvic inflammatory disease on page 195). The scar tissue may prevent ovulation, block the fallopian tubes so the ovum can't travel to the uterus, or otherwise prevent the reproductive organs from working properly. Hormone imbalances and certain diseases of the ovary can also prevent ovulation. Medical problems affecting the uterus and tubes can cause infertility, too.

In males, infertility is usually due to one of the following: too few sperm being produced, sperm that can't swim properly or are otherwise abnormal, or a blockage in the testicles or vas deferens which prevents the sperm from getting to the penis. These problems may be the result of a twisted vein in the testicle, hormonal imbalances, exposure to X-rays, drugs or other harmful substances, past infections, or other medical problems.

In many cases, infertility can be treated by medicines or surgery, but this isn't always possible.

How old is a woman before she's too old to have a baby?
Women stop having babies when they've gone through *menopause*. Menopause is the time in a woman's life when her ovaries stop producing a ripe ovum each month and she stops having her menstrual periods. It usually happens between the ages of forty-five and fifty-five, although it can happen earlier or later for some women.

As far as we know, the oldest woman who ever had

infertility (in-fer-TILL-uh-tee)
sterility (stuh-RILL-uh-tee)

a baby was a fifty-six-year-old grandmother from Glendale, California. Although her periods were coming only once in a while, the woman had not yet gone through menopause. She had sexual intercourse, and much to her surprise, she got pregnant. She gave birth to a normal, healthy baby.

Why are some babies girls and some boys?
The sex of the baby depends on the father's sperm. Some sperm have what scientists call an *"x"* chromosome, which means they are capable of uniting with an ovum and making a female baby. Other sperm have a *"Y"* chromosome, which means that they are capable of uniting with an ovum and making a male baby. If a *y*-factor sperm fertilizes the ovum, the baby will be a boy; if an *x*-factor sperm fertilizes the ovum, the baby will be a girl.

How long does pregnancy take?
Females are usually pregnant for about nine months; however, sometimes pregnancy can last a little longer or a little less than this. If the baby is born at only eight months or earlier, we say the baby is "premature." Many premature babies are perfectly normal and healthy; others need special medical care. If a baby is born very prematurely, before six months or so, its chances of surviving are much lower. If a pregnancy lasts much more than nine months, the doctor may give the woman

chromosome (CROW-moe-soam)

medication to make the baby come because it isn't healthy for the baby to stay in the uterus too long.

What happens when a baby is born?
When a baby is ready to be born, the mother goes into what we call labor. During labor, the muscles of the mother's uterus begin to contract rhythmically and the mother feels a cramping sensation. At first, the contractions aren't very strong and only come once in awhile. As labor continues, the contractions become stronger and stronger and come more often. At some point during labor or childbirth, the *amniotic sac*, the bag of fluids inside which the baby grows, breaks open, and the woman feels a gushing or leaking of fluid from her vagina. If the amniotic sac doesn't break on its own, the doctor will break it.

During labor, the opening of the cervix, the lower portion of the uterus that protrudes into the vagina, also begins to *dilate* (open up). When the cervix is fully dilated and the contractions are strong and regular, the force of the contractions begins to push the baby out of the uterus, through the cervix, through the vagina, and out the vaginal opening (see Illustration 41). Most babies are born head first, but some babies come out feet first or with some other part of the baby coming first. The average length of labor time for woman's first baby is about twelve to fourteen hours, and about seven hours for subsequent pregnancies.

For some women, labor and childbirth is very painful; for others there is little or no pain. But for most women, there is some discomfort, since the contractions have to be very strong in order to push the baby out. Some

amniotic (AM-knee-OT-ik)
dilate (DIE-late)

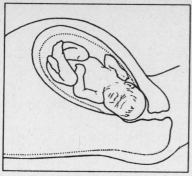

The cervix is fully dilated

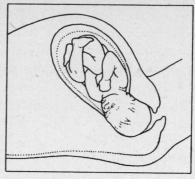

The baby's head moves into the vagina

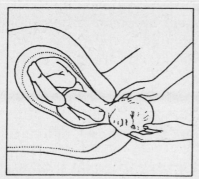

The baby's head comes out of the vagina

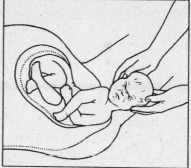

The baby's shoulders follow

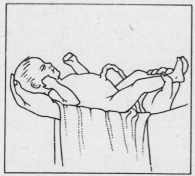

After the birth, the umbilical cord is clamped

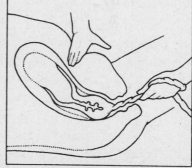

Afterward, the placenta is also pushed out of the uterus

Illustration 41. The Birth Process

women practice certain exercises before pregnancy and use breathing techniques during labor which help control the pain. If the pain is too intense, the woman may choose to have an anesthetic which numbs her from the waist down so she doesn't feel the pain.

Once labor has progressed to the point where the cervix is fully dilated (opened to about 4 inches), the "pushing stage" of labor begins. During this stage, the mother, if she hasn't been anesthetized, can bear down or push along with the contractions and help bring the baby out. Even if she can't help by pushing, the contractions alone are usually enough to push the baby out into the world. If not, the doctor can reach inside and help move the baby out.

This pushing stage usually lasts for one to three hours with a first pregnancy, and for about a half-hour with subsequent pregnancies, but it may be shorter or longer than this.

During the pushing stage, the baby begins to move out of the uterus and through the cervix into the vagina. Once the entire top of the baby's head is visible at the vaginal opening, things happen very quickly. It usually only takes a few more contractions to push the baby out entirely.

When a baby is born it has a cord, known as the *umbilical cord*, attached to its belly button. The other end of this cord is attached to the *placenta*. The placenta is a special organ that develops inside the uterus during pregnancy to bring blood and nourishment from the mother to the baby. The placenta usually comes out within a half-hour after the baby. The doctor then cuts

anesthetic (an-ess-THET-ik)
anesthetized (an-ESS-theh-TIZED)
umbilical (um-BILL-i-KUL)
placenta (pla-SEN-ta)

the cord and disposes of it and the placenta. The cord is cut within a couple of inches of the baby's belly button and is clamped or tied closed. By the time the baby is a few weeks old, the cord will have dried up and fallen off by itself.

After birth, the doctor or nurse checks the baby to make sure it's breathing property, and may clean it up a bit before giving it to its mother to hold. The boys and girls in my class get a big kick out of hearing about their own births. You might ask your mother to tell you about her labor with you.

What is a Cesarean section?

If for one reason or another, a baby can't be born in the normal way, the doctor does an operation called a *Cesarean* section, or C-section. The woman is anesthetized, so she can't feel anything from her waist down. The doctor makes an incision in her abdomen and uterus and removes the baby from her body by lifting it out through the incision. Afterwards, the incision is sewn shut. Babies born by C-section are usually perfectly healthy.

There are a number of reasons why a baby might have to be born by C-section. For example, labor may be taking so long that the baby is getting worn out and it's heartbeat is slowing down. Or the baby might be in a position that would make normal delivery difficult or impossible. The woman's cervix might not be dilating properly or her contractions might be too weak to push the baby out. For these or other reasons, the doctor might need to do a C-section.

Cesarean (si-ZARE-ee-en)

What is an embryo? What's a fetus?
After an ovum has been fertilized and has planted itself in the uterus, it begins the nine-month process of developing into a baby. For the first three months, it is referred to as an *embryo*. After three months, it is called a *fetus*.

What is a miscarriage? What is a stillbirth?
When an embryo or fetus dies, it is expelled from the mother's uterus and this is called *miscarriage*. Most miscarriages happen during the first three months of pregnancy, but they can happen later in pregnancy, too. Doctors aren't always sure why a miscarriage has happened, but usually the embryo or fetus has a defect or problem in its development that makes it impossible for it to survive. Having a miscarriage doesn't usually affect a woman's chances of having a normal baby in the future.

Stillbirth means that the baby is born dead. In some cases, the baby has died during the birth process; in other cases, the baby has died in the uterus shortly before birth. Sometimes the doctor can figure out why it happened; at other times it's a complete mystery. Fortunately, stillbirths and miscarriages after the third month of pregnancy are very rare. The vast majority of women have normal pregnancies and give birth to healthy babies.

What are birth defects and why do they happen?
Sometimes babies are born with medical problems such as blindness, brain damage, heart or lung problems,

embryo (EM-bree-oh)
fetus (FEE-tus)
miscarriage (MISS-care-ij)

deformed limbs, or other birth defects. Birth defects may be caused by defects in the ovum or sperm, inherited problems from the mother or father, the mother being exposed to harmful drugs or X-rays during pregnancy, a disease the mother has contracted during pregnancy, premature birth, or problems with the baby not getting enough oxygen right after birth. There are also other, less common causes, and sometimes the cause of a birth defect is not known. Fortunately, birth defects are very rare, and most babies are born completely healthy.

How do twins happen? How come twins don't always look alike? If a woman has twins, do they both come out at the same time?
Twins can happen in one of two ways: either there are two fertilized ova, or there is one fertilized ovum that splits in two (see Illustration 42).

Usually a woman's ovaries produce only one ripe ovum a month. Occasionally, though, a woman will produce two ripe ova at the same time. If both of these ova are fertilized and plant themselves in the lining of the uterus, the woman will have twins. Twins that grow from two separate ova, fertilized by two separate sperm, are called *fraternal* twins. With fraternal twins, one may be a boy and one a girl, or they may both be the same sex. They won't necessarily look alike.

The other type of twins is called *identical* twins. Identical twins happen when a fertilized ovum splits in two shortly after fertilization. No one knows why this happens. Twins that come from the same ovum and sperm look alike and are always the same sex.

When twins are born, one baby comes out first and the other comes out within a few minutes. In some cases, it takes more than a few minutes for the second

fraternal (frah-TUR-nul)

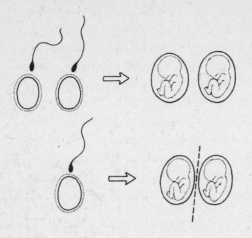

Sometimes a woman will produce two ripe ova the same month. If each of these ova is fertilized by sperm, the woman will have fraternal twins.

At other times, a sperm may fertilize a single ripe ovum. Then, after fertilization, the ovum splits into two, and the woman will have identical twins.

Illustration 42. Twins

twin to be born. There have even been cases where it took a whole day. But, usually, twins are born within a few minutes of each other.

What are Siamese twins?
Siamese twins are identical twins who are born with their bodies attached to each other in some way. Siamese twins happen when the fertilized ovum is splitting in two, making identical twins. But for some unknown reason, the split is not completed and the babies develop so that some parts of their bodies are joined together.

Identical twins are pretty rare. Siamese twins are even rarer. When Siamese twins do happen, they may be joined in a number of ways—at the feet, the shoulders, or the arms. When they are attached in such places, they are generally fairly easy to separate. A doctor can operate (usually shortly after the babies are born) and cut the babies apart. But sometimes it's not so easy. The babies may be joined at the head or chest or in such a way that cutting them apart would kill one or both of them. The parents may decide to have the operation done even though one baby will die. If the parents decide not to have the operation, or if it's not possible to operate without killing both babies, the twins spend their lives attached to each other.

What about triplets? What are the most babies a woman ever had at one time?

Triplets (three babies), quadruplets (four), quintuplets (five), sextuplets (six), septuplets (seven), and octuplets (eight) happen much less frequently than twins.

Whenever more than three babies are born at one time, the chances of all the babies surviving is lower. Because there are so many of them, they're smaller than normal babies, and they're usually born prematurely, that is, before they've had a chance to develop fully. As far as we know, the largest number of babies born at one time is twelve, but not all of them survived; the largest number that ever lived was eight, or possibly nine.

Nowadays, doctors have drugs, called *fertility drugs*, that they give to women who haven't been able to get pregnant because they don't ovulate. These drugs stimulate the ovaries and cause the woman to ovulate. The problem is that they can stimulate the ovaries so much that the woman produces not one but several ripe ova at the same time.

Birth Control

If two people want to have intercourse, but they don't want to become pregnant, they must use birth control. Birth control is also called *contraception* or family planning, and there are several different types or methods.

A lot of teens are getting pregnant these days—about 3,000 a day, or over a million each year. Experts estimate that four out of every ten of today's 14-year-old girls will have been pregnant at least once by the end of their teen years. So I spend a lot of time talking about birth control in my classes for older kids.

Even in my youngest classes, where most of the kids haven't yet started to go through puberty, I still spend at least some time talking about birth control. We think that starting to learn about contraception long before you might actually have a need for it is a good idea. That way, birth control becomes less mysterious, something you're used to hearing about as you grow older. When you do eventually become sexually active, you won't have to learn about birth control for the first time.

This section will help you start learning some of the basic facts about contraception. Of course, as you grow older, you'll need more information than is given here. Some of the books listed on pages 260–263 will help you learn more about contraception. If you are already sexually active or are thinking about having sex in the near future, you probably need more information than you'll find in this or any other book. You might want to visit your local Planned Parenthood clinic. They have special birth control classes for teens, and their nurses and doctors are experienced in helping young people

contraception (KON-treh-SEP-shen)

choose a method. Look under "Planned Parenthood" in the white pages, under "Family Planning" in the yellow pages, or call the information operator.

Of course, any family planning clinic or private doctor can help you learn about or obtain a method of birth control. And, anyone, regardless of their age, can get a prescription for or purchase any method of birth control. You don't need parental permission, and doctors are not required to notify your parents. So please don't hesitate to get the protection you need.

Methods of Birth Control

Most contraceptive methods currently in use work in one or more of the following ways: 1) by preventing ovulation, 2) by preventing fertilization, or 3) by altering the lining of the uterus so a fertilized ovum is prevented from growing there.

The most common methods are listed below. Most methods are "female" methods because they are employed by and affect the female, but the condom and male sterilization are "male" methods. Some methods require a doctor's prescription, but many (the sponge, spermicides, and condoms) can be purchased at drug stores, and even some grocery stores without a prescription.

Most of these methods are "temporary," meaning that once you stop using them, pregnancy is again possible. However, the last method listed—sterilization—is considered permanent because it is usually impossible for a person who's been sterilized to ever become pregnant again.

1. *Birth Control Pills:* A monthly series of hormone pills which protect against pregnancy as long as they are taken ac-

cording to schedule. However, forgetting to take even one pill may result in pregnancy. (Can be obtained only with a doctor's prescription.)

2. *The Intrauterine Device (IUD):* A soft plastic device which is inserted into the uterus by a doctor and which may be left in place up to several years, depending on the type used. The IUD should only be removed by a doctor—never by the woman herself. Because of safety hazards, the IUD is no longer manufactured in the US.

3. *The Diaphragm:* A soft rubber dome that is filled with a spermicide (sperm-killing chemical) and inserted into the vagina before sexual intercourse. If at least eight hours have passed since intercourse, the device can then be removed, cleaned, and stored for future use.

4. *The Cervical Cap:* Also used with spermicides, the cap is inserted, removed, and stored just like the diaphragm. The only difference is that the cap is smaller, shaped differently, covers only the cervix, and is held in place by suction.

5. *The Contraceptive Sponge:* Similar in size and shape to a powder puff, the sponge is moistened with water to release its spermicide and inserted into the top of the vagina before sex. It is used once and then thrown away.

6. *Spermicides:* May come in the form of creams or jellies which are used alone or with a cap or diaphragm: tablets, which dissolve when placed in the vagina; or aerosol foams, which are inserted into the vagina before sex by means of a special applicator.

7. *Condoms* ("rubbers"): A tube of thin rubber that fits over the erect penis like a glove over a finger. Held in place by a band of rubber at its lower edge, the condom traps semen inside. It is only used once and then thrown away. Most condoms come rolled up, in foil packets. If there isn't a "reservoir tip," one-half inch of space must be left at the top of the condom to allow room for the semen to collect.

intrauterine (In-trah-YOU-ter-in)
diaphragm (DIE-eh-FRAM)
condom (KON-dem)
spermicide (SPURM-eh-SIDE)

Otherwise, the semen could be forced down the sides of the penis and out the lower edge of the condom.

8. *The Rhythm Method:* Involves keeping track of the female's menstrual periods on a calendar and not having sex around the time of ovulation, when she is most likely to become pregnant. Because it is so difficult to guess when ovulation will occur (see pages 111–112), this is not a very effective method of birth control.

9. *Natural Family Planning (NFP):* An improvement on the rhythm method. Instead of just counting on a calendar, people who use NFP also keep charts of the female's daily body temperature and the type of mucous secreted by her cervix, which is a more accurate way of determining ovulation. Thus, NFP is much more effective than the rhythm method. Intercourse must be avoided on certain days with both rhythm and NFP.

10. *The Morning After Pill (MAP):* An emergency method which is only used when a female has had sex without the protection of birth control. The pills must be taken within 72 hours after sex in order to work. Because the dose of hormones is so high, this cannot be used as a regular method of birth control.

11. *Injectable Contraceptive:* A high dose of hormone injected into a female's body. The hormone is slowly released into the body. A single shot can prevent pregnancy for up to three months. (Not used in the United States, see page 185.)

12. *Abortion:* Used when people become pregnant but don't want to keep the baby or give it up for adoption. Abortions are usually done before the fourteenth week of pregnancy. An anesthetic is given and one end of a small suction tube is placed in the uterus. The other end of the tube is attached to a vacuum machine. The bloody menstrual lining and the developing pregnancy are then gently sucked out

sterilization (STARE-eh-leh-ZAY-shen)
abortion (uh-BORE-shen)

through the tube. Although abortions may be done up to the twenty-fourth week, these later abortions are more complicated and may have to be done in a hospital or clinic rather than at a doctor's office.

13. *Male or Female Sterilization:* An operation which in men is called *vasectomy* and in women *tubal ligation* or "tying the tubes." The vas deferens (the tube through which sperm travel from the testicles to the penis) or the fallopian tubes are cut, tied, sealed, or otherwise blocked off so pregnancy can't occur. Afterwards, the body keeps producing sperm and ova, but they are reabsorbed by the body.

Effectiveness

Although no birth control method is 100% effective, most of those listed here are highly effective, provided they are used correctly, *exactly according to instructions*. However, the rhythm method, the sponge, and spermicidal tablets, jellies, or creams used on their own (without a cap or a diaphragm) are the least effective. People who absolutely don't want to become pregnant should not use these methods.

You sometimes hear that methods like the pill and the IUD are more effective than condoms or diaphragms. Actually, people who use condoms and diaphragms (especially if they use them *with* foam or jelly) can get just as good results as people who use pills, *provided, of course, that they are used properly, each and every time a person has sex*.

Safety

Methods such as the diaphragm, cap, NFP, condoms, and foam are very safe because they don't cause any major side effects and rarely lead to any serious medical problems. Birth control pills are also considered safe,

vasectomy (vas-EK-teh-me)
ligation (leh-GAY-shen)

though not as safe as these other methods. The pill has reportedly caused heart attacks, strokes, and other serious medical problems in some users. However, these problems are not common and usually happen only in women who are over 35, who smoke cigarettes, or who have certain diseases (which is why doctors don't prescribe the pill for these women). Only *very* rarely do young, healthy, nonsmokers have problems with the pill, and most doctors consider the pill safe for these women.

Although most IUD users don't have problems, IUD manufacturers have been involved in many costly lawsuits brought by women who developed serious medical problems as a result of their IUDs. Therefore, the manufacturers in this country decided to stop making the IUD.

Some doctors are concerned that the injectable contraceptive might cause cancer or infertility in some women. Because of questions about the safety of this method, our government has not approved the injectable contraceptive for use in the United States, though it is available in many other countries.

Choosing the Right Method
Choosing a type of birth control involves weighing the relative effectiveness, convenience, and safety of each method. A couple's choice will also depend on many other factors including: the female's health, her age, the state of the couple's relationship, and whether they just want to "space" pregnancies or absolutely don't want to become pregnant. Most people use several different methods over the course of their lives.

Many young people begin by using a condom. The condom is easy to obtain and can protect against some sexually transmitted diseases (see pages 199–200). Later,

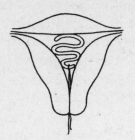

The IUD inside the uterus

The condom worn properly with room at the tip for semen to collect.

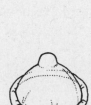

The condom

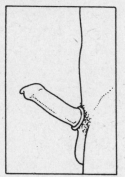

MON	TUES	WED	THUR	FRI	SAT	SUN
		1	2	3	4	5
6	7	8	~~9~~	~~10~~	~~11~~	~~12~~
~~13~~	~~14~~	15	16	17	18	19
20	21	22	23	24	25	26
27	28	29	30			

The rhythm method and Natural Family Planning (NFP) involve keeping track of the female's menstrual periods to determine when she will be ovulating.

Illustration 43. Types of birth control

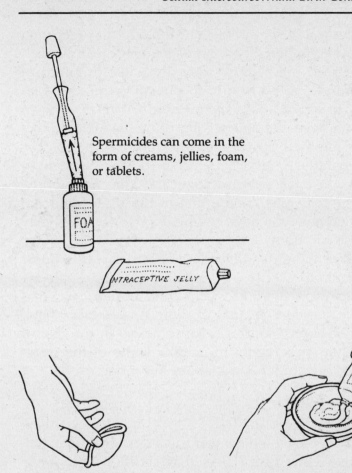

Spermicides can come in the
form of creams, jellies, foam,
or tablets.

The diaphragm

Applying spermicidal cream

The cervical cap

The contraceptive sponge

they may switch to one of the methods that require a doctor's prescription. Some couples prefer methods such as the IUD or pill because they don't like to interrupt their lovemaking by having to put on a condom, diaphragm, or cap or to use spermicides. However, women who don't have intercourse very often may choose one of these methods rather than the pill, which must be taken regularly, or an IUD, which is in place constantly. Women who are concerned about the side effects of the pill or the IUD may choose one of the safer methods. Men or women who have completed their families may choose sterilization.

The boys and girls in my class often ask lots of questions about birth control—more than we have space for here. However, there is one method in particular that they have questions about—abortion. As you may know, abortion is a very controversial topic, so in the rest of this section we're going to answer some of the questions that my students ask about abortion.

What's wrong with not using birth control and just having an abortion if you get pregnant?
Different people would answer this question somewhat differently. Some people feel that abortion is morally wrong, that it is the same as murder, and that it should be outlawed. They feel that a pregnant woman should have her baby and either keep the child or put it up for adoption. Since these people feel that abortion is morally wrong, they would, of course, feel that using abortion as a regular method of contraception (or, indeed, even once) is not okay.

Other people feel that abortion is a private matter between a woman and her doctor, and that a woman should have the right to decide what goes on inside her body, including whether or not she wants to have a baby. But even people who feel abortion is morally acceptable often feel that it's just not right or ethical for a person to rely on abortion as a regular method of birth control. They feel that abortion should only be used as a "back-up" measure when the regular method has failed to prevent pregnancy and the woman doesn't want to continue the pregnancy.

Aside from the moral and ethical reasons, there are also good medical reasons why people shouldn't have abortions whenever they become pregnant. If a woman didn't use contraception, she'd probably find herself getting pregnant at least once a year, if not more often. Having abortions this often could lead to serious medical problems.

How would a girl know whether or not she was pregnant?
Most females discover that they are pregnant because they fail to have their menstrual period at the expected time. Sore breasts and nausea are also early signs of pregnancy. There are many reasons other than pregnancy that could cause these symptoms, but pregnancy is the most common cause of missed periods in sexually active females. Anyone who thinks she might be pregnant should have a pregnancy test.

Standard pregnancy tests are done on a urine sample collected in the early morning. In order for the test to be accurate, at least fourteen days must have elapsed since the time of the expected menstrual period—that is, the female must be at least fourteen days "late" in getting her period. Standard pregnancy tests are available from private doctors or family planning clinics such as Planned Parenthood.

There are also tests that can detect pregnancy earlier, that is, before the female is fourteen days late in getting her period, but these are generally much more expensive. In addition, do-it-yourself pregnancy test kits are available at drug stores. If a person follows the directions exactly, these tests are quite reliable. However, it is possible to get a false test result. If the home pregnancy test indicates a female isn't pregnant, but she still doesn't get her period, or she has other signs of pregnancy, or if she feels unsure about the test results, she should have a test done at a doctor's office or clinic.

What if the test shows that you are pregnant?

If pregnancy occurs, there are three choices: 1) continuing the pregnancy and keeping the baby, 2) continuing the pregnancy but giving the child up for adoption, and 3) abortion. If you are not certain which is the best choice for you, the doctor at the place where you got your pregnancy test can refer you to a counselor who will help you decide. Regardless of what decision you make, you have the right to sympathetic counseling and to complete information about each of the choices available. Even if you feel certain about your decision, you may find it helpful to discuss your decision with a member of your family or a counselor.

Does a girl need her parent's permission to get an abortion? How much does it cost? Where can you get an abortion?

A girl doesn't need her parent's permission in order to have an abortion, regardless of her age. Abortions can be done in doctor's offices, hospitals, or clinics. They usually cost anywhere from $150 and $350, depending on the type of abortion and when it is done. If a girl can't afford to pay for an abortion, she can usually arrange for the government to pay for it. Planned Parenthood clinics can provide abortion services or referrals, as well as information about free or low-cost abortions. State or county welfare offices can also provide this information (ask the information operator for the state or county Welfare Department or the Department of Human and Social Services).

After we've talked about intercourse, pregnancy and childbirth, and birth control in class, we usually move on to the topic of sexually transmitted diseases, and then to other sexual health issues. There isn't any special reason why we move from one topic to the next in this order, but since that's usually how it happens, in the next chapter we'll discuss these topics in pretty much the same order that we do in class.

CHAPTER 10

Sexually Transmitted Diseases, AIDS, and Other Sexual Health Issues

One day not long ago, the kids in my fifth-grade class and I were going through the class question box. I pulled out a folded scrap of paper which had these two questions written on it:

> What is BD?
> What is Ben Aerial's disease and what does it have to do with sex?

At first, I didn't have a clue as to what these questions were about. I just stood there, staring at the paper and mumbling to myself: "BD? . . . Ben Aerial? . . . like the antenna on a television set? . . . *Ben Aerial's disease??* . . . What in the world???"

Then all of a sudden I realized what had happened: The student who wrote these questions had apparently overheard some people talking and thought they were saying *BD* when it was really *VD* they were talking about. He wanted to find out about *venereal disease* (not Ben Aerial's disease!), which is a group of diseases people can get from having sex.

In the first section of this chapter, we'll be talking about these diseases. However, because VD is a sort of old-fashioned term, we'll be using the more modern term, "sexually transmitted diseases," or STDs.

You may notice that we haven't included AIDS, an STD that's been in the news a lot lately, in the section on STDs. That's because AIDS is different from the other STDs in several important ways; therefore, we decided to discuss AIDS in a separate section of its own.

The AIDS section follows the STD section. In addition, there are two other sections in this chapter that deal with health problems related to the sex organs or sexual activity. We hope this chapter helps answer any questions you may have about these sexual health issues.

Sexually Transmitted Diseases (STDs)

Each year more than a million teenagers in the United States develop an STD. Since these diseases are usually transmitted sexually, kids who haven't started having sex yet don't really need to worry about STDs. Still, we think it never hurts to start learning about them while you're still young. Besides, kids are often curious about this topic, so even in my classes for younger kids, I spend some time talking about STDs.

In this section we'll be explaining the basic facts about STDs. If, however, you'd like more information than is given here, you'll find some helpful books in the Further Reading list in the back of this book. You can also call the National VD Hotline (see page 201) for information about STDs.

Symptoms

There are more than twenty different types of STDs. Although each type has its own particular symptoms, generally speaking, STDs cause the following kinds of symptoms:

- An unusual discharge from the penis or vagina.
- Itching, burning, redness, rashes, lumps, bumps, or sores in, on, or around the sex organs.
- Pain or tenderness in the sex organs, the genital area, or the lower abdomen.
- Burning or pain when urinating, or a frequent need to urinate.

These symptoms can also be caused by diseases that aren't sexually transmitted, but any sexually active person who develops these symptoms needs to see a doctor in order to be tested for STDs, and if necessary, treated.

It is possible to have an STD but not have any symptoms or have only mild, temporary symptoms that clear up on their own, without treatment. Nonetheless, the germs may still be in the body, which means the person is still capable of passing the disease to other people.

Types of STDs

Syphilis is an STD that was a dreaded disease back before antibiotics had been discovered. The germs would spread from the sex organs to the brain, heart, lungs, and other organs, causing insanity and/or death. Nowadays, though, syphilis can be treated with antibiotics before it has a chance to spread.

Gonorrhea and *chlamydia* are two very common STDs which are serious problems for females because, unlike males, females often don't have any symptoms and, therefore, don't seek treatment. Thus, the germs may

syphilis (SIF-eh-lis)
gonorrhea (GONE-ah-REE-uh)
chlamydia (KLUH-mid-ee-uh)

remain in the vagina. Then, weeks, months, or even years later, the germs may move upwards, spreading the infection to the uterus, fallopian tubes, and ovaries. Infection of these organs, known as *pelvic inflammatory disease* (PID), can be a very serious type of STD. It often requires a hospital stay, and in some cases, it may be necessary to operate and remove the infected organs. Even if there are no symptoms or only mild ones, PID can seriously damage these organs, causing infertility or life-long recurrences of the infection, as well as other major health problems.

Genital warts and *genital herpes*, which are also very common, are both caused by viruses. Here again, these STDs can be especially serious for females because these viruses sometimes lead to cervical cancer. Herpes can also cause miscarriages, premature births, and other problems during childbirth and pregnancy. In fact, herpes, whose chief symptom is painful, blister-like sores, can be serious for both males and females because, unlike other STDs, herpes is incurable. Once you get it, the virus remains in your body for the rest of your life. But this doesn't mean you'll always have the sores, or are always capable of passing the disease on to others. After a few weeks, the viruses retreat deep into the body. The sores disappear and the person is no longer capable of infecting others. However, the viruses usually surface from time to time, causing new outbreaks of the sores and other symptoms. During these outbreaks, and for a time before and after, the person is again capable of passing the virus on to his or her sex partner.

Not all STDs are this serious. For instance, *tricho-moniasis* (trich or TV), *candidiasis* (yeast infections), and

herpes (HER-peez)
trichomoniasis (TRICK-o-moan-EYE-uh-sis)
candidiasis (CAN-di-DIE-uh-sis)

Gardnerella (Hemophilus) can cause bothersome symptoms, but they rarely, if ever, lead to major medical problems. In fact, although males may pass these infections to their female sex partners, they themselves don't usually develop any symptoms. The same is true of *nonspecific vaginitis*, an STD that affects females. "Vaginitis" means inflammation of the vagina and "nonspecific" means the doctor can't find any specific germ that's causing the infection.

Nonspecific urethritis (NSU) is another infection that is often (though not always) transmitted sexually. "Urethritis" means inflammation of the urethra and "nonspecific" means the doctor can't pinpoint a specific germ that is causing the urinary symptoms. NSU is more common in males than in females. Although NSU can lead to cystitis (infections of the bladder) and other more serious kidney or urinary tract infections, it is usually treated before these problems occur. Thus, NSU isn't considered as serious as some of the other STDs.

Pubic lice, or "crabs," is perhaps the least serious of all the STDs, though it's certainly no fun having them. The lice are tiny, crab-like, bloodsucking insects that can be found in the pubic hair, head hair, and sometimes the eyelashes. Their bite causes intense itching that is often worse at night. Getting rid of lice involves repeated shampoos with a special lotion, and dry cleaning or boiling all bed linen, undergarments, and any other infected clothing (or stuffing them in a plastic bag for two weeks) to make sure all the lice are dead.

Gardnerella (GARD-ner-ELL-uh)
Hemophilus (he-MOF-eh-lus)
vaginitis (VAJ-en-NI-tis)
urethritis (YOUR-rith-RYE-tis)
cystitis (sis-TIE-tis)

How STDs Are Spread

Most STDs are caused by germs that can only survive in the moist, mucous membranes of the human body, that is, in places like the penis, vulva, vagina, rectum, mouth, or throat. Most of the germs die almost immediately when exposed to air. However, certain STD germs, such as trichs, can survive for several hours on objects like toilet seats or towels. But, for the most part, STD germs die soon after leaving the human body.

Because these germs generally survive only in mucous membranes, STDs are usually transmitted (spread) when an infected person's mucous membranes come in contact with another person's mucous membranes. This kind of membrane-to-membrane contact usually only happens during some form of sexual activity. However, it's not necessary for a male to ejaculate in order to pass the disease to his sex partner; any type of membrane-to-membrane contact can spread the disease. It is also possible to spread certain STDs from one part of the body to another with the fingers. For instance, touching a herpes sore and then touching your eye could lead to an eye infection (which could cause blindness). And touching an STD sore or discharge and then touching another person's mucous membranes could also spread the disease.

STDs can be also be transmitted in other nonsexual ways. For instance, certain STDs can be passed from an infected mother to her baby before or during birth. This can be very serious for the baby and may cause blindness, mental retardation, or other birth defects.

Candidiasis (yeast infections) can also be spread in nonsexual ways. Improper wiping after a bowel movement may bring yeasts from a female's rectum into her vagina. In addition, yeasts normally live in some females' vaginas, though the natural acidity of the vagina keeps them in check. However, taking antibiotics, using birth control pills, being pregnant, or having diabetes may make the vagina less acid, allowing the yeasts to reproduce wildly and cause a vaginal discharge and other symptoms.

Although PID is usually the result of sexually transmitted germs moving up into the female pelvic organs, operations, abortions, and childbirth can also lead to PID. Trich, Gardnerella, nonspecific vaginitis, nonspecific urethritis, and pubic lice can also be transmitted in nonsexual ways.

Though STDs can be spread in these nonsexual ways, most cases of STDs are the result of sexual activity. We should, however, mention that you can't get STDs from masturbating by yourself, from sitting clothed on someone else's lap, from a swimming pool or hot tub, or in any way other than the ones explained here or on the following pages.

The questions and answers in the following pages may help you understand more about STDs.

I heard that if you get a cold sore on your lip, it means you have herpes. Is this true?

In order to understand the answer to this question, you need to understand first that there are different types of herpes viruses and that they cause different kinds of diseases. Chicken pox, for instance, is caused by a herpes virus. The common cold sore, or fever blister, is also caused by another herpes virus, known as herpes simplex, type I (HSV-1), which results in blister-like sores in and around the mouth. Genital herpes is caused by a similar but different herpes virus, known as herpes virus, type II (HSV-2), which usually causes blister-like sores on or around the genital (sex) organs.

Having a cold sore only means that you "have herpes"

in the sense that someone with chicken pox has herpes, that is, you have an infection caused by one of the herpes viruses. Having a cold sore *does not* mean you have the sexually transmitted disease known as genital herpes or just plain "herpes," as it is sometimes called.

Can you get an STD from kissing?

As a general rule, the answer to this question is no. However, there are some exceptions. Having oral-genital sex with someone who has a syphilis or herpes sore in his or her genital area could cause the sore to appear on your lip or mouth. Or, if you kissed a person who had one of these sores on the mouth or lip, you could get herpes or syphilis. (This is why it's not a good idea to kiss someone who has a sore on the lip, or to have oral-genital sex with a person who has a sore in the genital area.)

The only other exception is that it might be possible to get certain STDs from French-kissing (deep, open-mouth kissing where one or both people put their tongues in the other person's mouth). For instance, people can get gonorrhea germs in the back of the throat from oral-genital sex. So, if you French-kissed such a person, it would be possible to get the infection this way.

Can you get an STD from a toilet seat, a drinking glass, a towel, a wash cloth, or other object?

Except for STDs like pubic lice, which can live for a few days outside the human body, or trichs, which can survive for a number of hours, most STD germs die almost instantly when they leave the mucous membranes and are exposed to air. So, generally speaking, the answer to this question is no. In fact, in order to get an STD from a toilet seat, you'd have to put your mucous membranes in contact with the seat *immediately* after the seat had come in contact with the discharge or the mucous membranes of a person who had an STD. This, of course, isn't very likely to happen. It would be possible to get STD from an object like a drinking glass, towel, or wash cloth if it had *just* been used by a person with an STD sore, or an STD discharge. But, as a general rule, people don't get STDs from objects.

How can a person tell if he or she has an STD?
There are special medical tests to determine whether or not a person has an STD, and if so what kind. One way people find out that they have an STD is that they develop symptoms like the ones described above. The symptoms lead the person to see a doctor who tests him or her to see if the symptoms are being caused by an STD.

Because a person can have an STD without knowing it and because untreated STDs can lead to serious health problems, it is *vitally important* that anyone who's had contact with an infected person seek medical attention *right away*, regardless of whether or not they have symptoms. And people diagnosed as having an STD must inform *all* their sexual partners, so these people can be tested and, if necessary, treated. Even if the sexual partners don't have any symptoms, they must still be tested and treated.

What should you do if you think you might have an STD?
You should go straight to a doctor or clinic. Private doctors treat STDs and most Planned Parenthood clinics also provide free or low-cost STD testing and treatment. You can also get free testing and treatment from your county Health Department.

You don't need your parents' permission to be tested or treated, and no one will inform your parents that you have been. Doctors and the people who work at clinics are used to dealing with young people who have STDs. You don't need to feel embarrassed or ashamed to go for testing.

Even if you don't have symptoms, but think you may have had contact with an infected person, it's very important that you be tested. Even if your symptoms have disappeared, the germs could still be in your body causing damage, and you could still pass the infection to others.

Most STDs can be treated quite easily—usually with antibiotics—*provided they are treated right away*. But, if they go undetected and untreated, they can cause lasting damage to the body.

If you have questions regarding testing or treatment (or any other questions about STDs) you can call the National VD Hotline, 800-227-8922. This is a toll-free number, so there's no charge for the call and it won't appear on your phone bill. The call is confidential and you don't have to give your name, so don't hesitate to call.

Is there anything you can do to prevent getting an STD?
There are a number of things you can do to help prevent or at least cut down on your chances of getting an STD. First of all, personal hygiene is very important. You should wash your genitals every day and wear clean cotton underwear. Avoid deodorants, perfumes, and strong or scented soaps as they can irritate and dry out the genital skin, making it more susceptible to infection. Avoid synthetic underwear, tight jeans, and other tight clothing because they cut down on air flow and keep the genital area damp, making it more susceptible to infection. Females should always wipe from front to back, away from the vagina, when going to the bathroom, to avoid transferring germs from the rectum to the vagina.

Using condoms will help prevent STDs, though they do not offer 100% protection. Spermicides have also been shown to reduce the chances of developing STDs. The cervical cap and the diaphragm also cut down the chances of a female developing certain types of STDs. But none of these methods offers 100% protection.

Above all, never have sex with a person who has STD symptoms—that is, unusual discharges, or rashes or sores on or around their sex organs. If you or your sexual partner currently has an STD, do not have any form of sexual contact again until the doctors says it's safe to do so.

Waiting until you're older before you start to have sex may also cut down on your chances of getting an STD. People who start their sex lives at an earlier age generally have a greater number of sexual partners in the course of their lives (and hence more STDs) than people who wait until they're older.

Choosing your sexual partners carefully is also important in preventing sexually transmitted diseases. If you don't know your sexual partner well, you don't know if that person is the type who'd inform you if he or she did develop symptoms later on. For this reason, it is always a good idea to use a condom when you start having sex with a new partner, when you are having sex with someone who has other sexual partners, or if you yourself have more than one partner.

STDs can lead to serious health problems, especially for women, so taking the preventive measures and precautions described above is very important.

AIDS

The letters in the word AIDS stand for Acquired Immune Deficiency Syndrome. It is a relatively new disease. The first cases in this country were discovered in 1981. AIDS is considered an STD because it is most often spread through sexual intercourse. But because AIDS is different from other STDs and because it is such a serious disease, we decided to discuss AIDS in a special section of its own.

Scientists believes AIDS is caused by a virus. The AIDS virus attacks the immune system, the body's built-in defense against disease. The immune system keeps us healthy by destroying many of the disease-causing germs that get into our bodies and helps us to recover if we do become ill. The AIDS virus prevents the immune system from doing its job properly, so people with AIDS may become deathly ill from diseases that other people would recover from quite easily. People with AIDS may also develop certain rare, life-threatening illnesses that people with normal, undamaged immune systems would never have gotten in the first place. The AIDS virus can also infect the brain, causing serious and deadly brain diseases.

How Is AIDS Transmitted?

You may have heard all sorts of rumors about how AIDS is spread. If so, it's important to remember that the AIDS virus doesn't live *in* the air or *on* the things we touch, the way cold or flu viruses do. This means you can't get AIDS from what doctors call "casual contact"—that is, from coughs or sneezes, from eating food, from touching objects or people, or from being around an infected person. You can't get AIDS from normal everyday activities such as working at a job, attending school, using a public bathroom, taking a bath or shower,

acquired (eh-CHOIR-ed)
immune (eh-MUNE)
deficiency (dee-FISH-n-see)
syndrome (SIN-drome)

swimming in a pool, sitting in a hot tub, eating in a restaurant, shaking hands, using headphones, having someone whisper in your ear or breathe on you, hugging someone, or drinking from a glass or water fountain.

Scientists know that AIDS can't be spread through casual contact because, if it could be, there'd be many, many doctors, nurses, family members, and other people living with or caring for AIDS patients who would have come down with the disease. All of the people who've gotten the disease in this country have gotten it in one of the following ways:

1. *Sexual Intercourse:* Most cases of AIDS are spread through some type of sexual intercourse. Many people have the mistaken idea that infected females can't pass the disease to their male sexual partners, but this isn't true. People of either sex can pass the disease to their sex partners.

2. *IV Needles:* The second most common way in which AIDS is passed is through sharing needles used to inject illegal IV drugs such as heroin (smack), cocaine, "speed," or other "hard" drugs. When people use IV (intravenous) needles to "shoot up" (inject such drugs), some of their blood is drawn back up into the needle. Sometimes it's only a small amount of blood, too small to be seen. But, if a person uses a needle that has even a tiny amount of blood from an infected person, he or she can get AIDS.

   You can't, however, get AIDS from an injection given by a doctor, nurse, or health worker. These people use disposable needles or ones that have been properly sterilized, so there's no danger of getting AIDS.

   We should also mention the fact that there have been a very small number of cases in which a doctor, nurse, or other health care worker developed AIDS as a result of accidentally sticking themselves with a needle while drawing blood from or giving an injection of medicine to an AIDS patient.

3. *Blood Transfusions:* Although it is less common than #1 or #2 above, it is also possible for a person to get AIDS from

having a transfusion of blood or blood products. Such transfusions are sometimes given before, during, or after an operation if a person has lost too much blood. People who
have certain medical problems, such as hemophilia (a disease in which the blood does not clot properly so that even
a small cut or bruise can result in uncontrollable bleeding),
may also be given transfusions. We now have a special test
to make sure the blood or blood products used in transfusions are not infected with the AIDS virus. So nowadays,
there is very little chance of a person becoming infected in
this way. But those who had transfusions between 1976 and
1985 (when the test became available) could have gotten
AIDS if infected blood or blood products were used in the
transfusion. *A person can't, however, get AIDS from donating
(giving) blood.*

We should also mention that there have been at least
three cases where a nurse or other health care worker developed AIDS after accidentally spilling infected blood from
an AIDS patient onto an open cut, sore, or break in the
skin. This was, in effect, the same as a blood transfusion,
for it allowed viruses from the infected blood to travel directly into the health care worker's bloodstream.

4. *Pregnant Woman to Infant:* An infected pregnant woman can
pass the AIDS virus into her unborn baby's bloodstream
because the mother and the developing baby share the same
blood. This is not, however, a common way of passing AIDS
at the present time; less than 1% of AIDS cases in the United
States as of 1987 were caused in this way.

What all this means is that if you haven't started
having sex yet *and* you have never used illegal IV drugs
and you have never had a blood transfusion, there's
just no way you could have the disease. So, you can
relax. But even if you are sexually active, there are
things you can do to protect yourself from AIDS. Whatever you do, don't let fear keep you from learning the
facts you need to know.

hemophilia (HE-moe-FEEL-ee-ah)

Exposure, Infection, and Disease

Young people often want to know if everyone who comes in contact with the AIDS virus actually gets AIDS. Just as people don't get colds or flu every time they come in contact with a cold or flu virus, neither does everyone who comes into contact with the AIDS virus get AIDS.

However, a lot of the confusion about AIDS stems from the fact that most people don't really understand the difference between coming in *contact* with a virus, becoming *infected* with the virus, and actually *developing* a viral disease. The table below gives some definitions we think are helpful in terms of understanding how any virus, including the AIDS virus, "works."

> *Phase 1: Exposure.* Exposure means a person has come in actual physical contact with the virus. Exposure doesn't necessarily lead to infection, but it *may* lead to phase 2, infection.
>
> *Phase 2: Infection.* Infection means the virus has actually moved inside some of the cells of the person's body. Any infected person is capable of infecting others. But being infected doesn't necessarily mean the person will develop symptoms. However, infection *may* lead to phase 3, disease.
>
> *Phase 3: Disease.* Disease means the person has not only been exposed and infected, but has actually come down with symptoms. In such cases, we say the person "has" the disease.

We don't know how many of the people *exposed* to the virus will actually become infected. Nor do we know how many of those *infected* will actually come down with AIDS. At first experts thought that only about 20% to 30% of those infected would eventually develop symptoms. But recent studies suggest that this percentage may be much higher. Many experts are now afraid that as many as 90% of those infected may eventually come down with AIDS or ARC, a related disease (see page 209).

Important Facts About AIDS

The following facts are important for anyone who hopes to understand AIDS:

- AIDS has spread at an alarming rate. In 1981, 321 cases of AIDS were reported in the U.S. By the end of 1986, 40,000 Americans had been diagnosed as having AIDS. By 1991, experts estimate that the total number of cases will have reached anywhere from 250,000 to 750,000 (or more).
- As of 1987, about 25,000 Americans have died of AIDS.
- The AIDS virus belongs to a certain category or type of rare virus. Scientists have never found a cure for any of the diseases caused by this class of virus, so they don't expect to find a cure for AIDS any time soon. (Some are afraid that a cure may never be found.) So far, no one has ever recovered from AIDS.
- Some people infected by the AIDS virus develop symptoms within a few months; others don't develop symptoms for a number of years. It is not uncommon for the symptoms to take five years or even longer to show up.
- Experts estimate that as of 1987, two million Americans have been infected with the AIDS virus (though many of these people are not aware of this fact, since they haven't yet developed symptoms).

These facts explain why government leaders, doctors, health officials, as well as many other people, are so worried about AIDS.

The questions and answers on the following pages will help you understand more about AIDS. However, if you are a drug user, if you're already having sex, or if you're even thinking about it, you need more detailed information than we have room for in this book. We hope you'll read the book on AIDS that we wrote especially for young people like you. It's called *Lynda Madaras Talks to Teens About AIDS* (Newmarket Press, 1988). It's a short book, but it gives you all the information you need to protect yourself from AIDS. Reading it could literally save your life! You might also want to send away for some of the free pamphlets listed on 260–263 of this book, or look at some of the books and videos listed there.

The material in this section is based on the most up-to-date information that was available at the time this book went to press. But scientists are making new discoveries all the time. You can get the most recent, accurate information by calling the Public Health Service AIDS Hotline, toll-free, at 800-342-AIDS. There is no charge for the call. It won't appear on your phone bill and you don't need to give your name. A trained counselor will answer any questions you may have.

What kinds of symptoms does AIDS cause?
Some people don't have any symptoms at first, and they look and feel completely healthy. For others, the disease may begin with one or more of the following symptoms: swollen glands, extreme tiredness, loss of appetite; sudden and unplanned weight loss, night sweats, skin rashes, fevers, headaches, diarrhea, and white spots or a white coating on the tongue. Many of these symptoms can also be caused by more common diseases, including colds and flu. The difference is that AIDS symptoms tend to last much longer than you'd normally expect.

As the immune system breaks down, other diseases develop and cause other symptoms. For instance, many AIDS patients get a rare form of cancer that causes pink, brown, or purple lumps on the inside or outside of the body. Some get a rare pneumonia which causes coughing, chest pain, and difficulty in breathing. Some get brain diseases and have symptoms such as personality changes, loss of memory, and other signs of mental illness.

Some people with AIDS get sick and stay sick until they die. Others have periods of being quite healthy, followed by periods of sickness, then recovery, then sickness, and so on. Eventually, though, they are no longer able to recover.

What is ARC? How is ARC different from AIDS?
ARC stands for <u>A</u>IDS-<u>R</u>elated <u>C</u>omplex. Like people with AIDS, people with ARC have become infected with the AIDS virus and have developed symptoms. ARC symptoms tend to be less serious, though in some cases ARC patients may be quite ill and may even die. Experts estimate that 10% to 20% of the people with ARC will eventually develop AIDS.

Is there a test for AIDS?
Scientists hope to have a test that could detect the AIDS virus by the end of 1988. Until then we only have the AIDS antibody test. *Antibodies* are substances that the immune system makes to try and destroy viruses or other disease-causing organisms. Different antibodies are made for each different type of germ. The AIDS antibody test involves taking a sample of the person's blood and studying it in a scientific laboratory to see if there are any AIDS antibodies. If there are, the test is positive. If there aren't, the test is negative.

But the AIDS antibody test only tells us whether the person has AIDS antibodies. It doesn't tell us whether the person has actually become infected with the virus or whether he or she will eventually develop symptoms. So, until we have a better test, people with positive antibody tests should not have babies or do anything else that might spread the disease to others.

If the antibody test is negative, doesn't this show that the person hasn't been infected with the virus?

Not necessarily. It usually takes four to eight weeks, and sometimes as long as six months, for a person to produce enough antibodies to show up on the test. So, if a person became infected and had the test right away, before the antibodies had enough time to build up, that person might have a negative antibody test, even though he or she really was infected. Therefore, if you wanted to be certain you didn't have the virus, you would have to make sure you didn't do anything that could possibly expose you to the virus for six months before you had the test.

If it can take years to develop symptoms, how can scientists be sure that AIDS can't be passed through casual contact? Isn't it possible that people living with or caring for AIDS patients really have gotten the disease through casual contact, but that it just hasn't shown up yet?

These are good questions and ones that many people ask. Although it's true that it can take many years for the symptoms to show up, the antibodies show up fairly quickly.

Scientists have given repeated antibody tests over a period of many months, and even years, to thousands of family members, nurses, doctors, and others who have had casual contact with AIDS patients. Except for those who had used IV drugs, had blood transfusions, or had sex with an infected person, *none* of these people have had positive antibody tests. Therefore, scientists are sure the disease can't be spread through casual contact.

Could you get AIDS from a mosquito bite or from some other kind of insect bite?

No. For one thing, blood-sucking insects usually wait twenty-four hours or longer between feedings, and the

AIDS virus would die long before this. Also, insects only withdraw blood. They don't inject blood into a person. Besides, if mosquitoes could spread the disease, we'd be seeing an unusually high number of AIDS cases in areas of the country where there are mosquitoes, and this isn't the case. There was a rumor about people in a town in Florida getting AIDS from mosquito bites, but it turned out not to be true. Scientists are quite certain that you can't get AIDS from insect bites.

I heard that infected people can have the virus in their saliva and tears, so couldn't the disease be passed through contact with these body fluids? If you were bitten by an infected person would you get AIDS? Can you get AIDS from kissing? How about French kissing? We lumped these questions together because they have similar answers. It is true that the AIDS virus has been found in the saliva and tears of some AIDS patients.* However, this doesn't mean that AIDS can be transmitted by contact with tears or by a simple kiss. If people could get AIDS in these ways, there would be a lot more cases of AIDS among family members and health workers. Moreover, even when infected people do have the virus in their saliva, the actual number of viruses is very small. So, even if a person did get some saliva from kissing an infected person, there wouldn't be enough viruses absorbed through the mucous membranes of the mouth to cause the person to become infected.

Scientists are not entirely certain what would happen if a person who had an open sore or cut on the mouth

---

* Some kids in my classes have the mistaken idea that this means that the body is getting rid of the virus or that people could somehow spit or cry the viruses out of their bodies altogether. Neither of these things is true. Tears and saliva don't rid the body of the viruses. There will still be more viruses in the blood, constantly reproducing and making more viruses.

kissed an infected person or if a person were bitten by an infected person. Open sores or cuts and bites that break the skin would allow any virus in infected saliva to travel directly into the person's bloodstream, so scientists can't rule out the possibility of the disease being passed in these ways. However, we do know that there have been cases of people being bitten by AIDS patients, and that none of the people bitten have become infected. Nor do we know of anyone with an open mouth sore or cut getting AIDS from kissing. (Still, it's never a good idea to kiss someone while you have a sore or cut on your mouth—not just because of AIDS, but also because of other germs.)

There aren't any known cases of people getting AIDS from French kissing ("open mouth" kissing where one or both people put their tongues in each other's mouth). However, there are certain cells that can be found deep in the back of the throat that can carry the AIDS virus. So here again, scientists can't say that it's 100% impossible to get AIDS in this way.

Can people get AIDS from oral-genital sex?
Scientists can't be sure because the people who've gotten AIDS have usually had not just oral-genital sex, but other types of sex as well. Therefore, no one knows if oral-genital sex alone would transmit the disease. However, we know that the virus can live in vaginal secretions and in the semen of infected males, so most experts feel that oral-genital sex probably can transmit the disease.

Is it true that in this country the majority of persons with AIDS are male homosexuals or bisexuals, and male and female heterosexuals who use illegal IV drugs? Does this mean heterosexuals who don't use drugs and haven't had blood transfusions don't really need to worry about AIDS?
In order to understand the answer to these questions,

you need to know that a male *homosexual* is a person who has sex with other males; a male *bisexual* is a person who has sex with other males and also with females; a *heterosexual* is a person who has sex with people of the opposite sex. (All of this is explained in more detail in the next chapter, so you might want to jump ahead to pages 240–243 before you read the answer to these questions.)

The answer to the first question above is yes. The majority of cases of AIDS reported in this country have occurred among male homosexuals and bisexuals, or among male or female heterosexuals who use IV drugs.

However, the answer to the second question is no. Despite what some people think, AIDS is not a "homosexual" or "drug-users" disease. In fact, in other parts of the world, such as Africa, AIDS is more common among heterosexuals than among homosexuals, and it is equally common among males and females. Even though the majority of cases in this country so far have occurred among homosexuals, bisexuals and drug users, this *does not* mean the disease will continue to be confined to these groups. In the future, experts expect to see larger numbers of heterosexuals who've never had transfusions and who don't use IV drugs getting AIDS. Indeed, many such people have already been infected with the virus, but because it can take so long for symptoms to develop, we haven't yet seen large numbers of such people coming down with AIDS. Just about anyone who is sexually active needs to be concerned about AIDS and to take steps to protect against the virus.

homosexual (hoe-moe-SEC-shoe-ul)
bisexual (bye-SEC-shoe-ul)
heterosexual (HET-er-oh-SEC-shoe-ul)

What do people mean when they say, "Nowadays, when you have sex with someone, you're not only having sex with that person, but with everyone he or she has had sex with and those people's sex partners, too?"

They mean that even though your sex partner isn't a male homosexual or bisexual, isn't a drug user, and isn't someone who's ever had a blood transfusion, he or she may have had sex with someone who is, or that person's previous sex partners may have had sex with such a person. In either case, your sex partner may have gotten the virus, and even though he or she may not have symptoms, he or she could pass the virus on to you.

How can I protect myself from getting AIDS?

When young people ask us this question, the first thing we tell them is: DON'T USE ILLEGAL IV DRUGS! Don't use them even once. In fact, stay away from all illegal drugs, because using these drugs increases the chances that a person will get "hooked" on drugs and will eventually go on to use IV drugs. (Those who do use IV drugs should *never* share needles.) Don't have sex with anyone who uses these drugs or with someone who has sex with drug users.

The second thing we tell young people who ask this question is that AIDS is mainly a sexually transmitted disease. Therefore, abstinence, that is, waiting until you're older or until you're married before you have sex, is, of course, the most effective way of preventing AIDS. We also remind young people not to make the mistake of thinking that having sexual intercourse is the only way to have a deep, meaningful, pleasurable, and romantic sexual experience with someone else. Hugging, touching, kissing, and other activities that don't involve the exchange of body fluids are "safe" ways of expressing and sharing sexual feelings.

Finally, if you're going to have sex, USE CONDOMS.

Some young people have a hard time believing that this advice applies to them. They don't think that anyone they'd be having sex with could possibly have the virus, so they don't see why they need to use condoms. But nowadays just about anyone could have the virus. Unless your sex partner answers "no" to the following questions and you're *sure* he or she is telling the truth, you *must* use condoms:

1. Have you ever had a transfusion of blood or blood products?
2. Have you ever used illegal IV drugs?
3. Have you ever before had any type of sexual intercourse (including oral-genital sex)?
4. Will you be using IV drugs or having intercourse with anyone else during the course of your sexual relationship?

It's important to remember that just as condoms may not be 100% effective in preventing pregnancy, they also may not be 100% efective in preventing AIDS. For example, condoms that are too old or are stored improperly may break or leak. Moreover, people don't always use them properly. If you're not absolutely certain that you know how to buy, use, and store condoms, you should contact your local Planned Parenthood or the AIDS hotline (800-342-AIDS). If you don't know the facts about condoms or if you feel too shy or embarrassed to talk to a potential sex partner about condoms, we suggest you read our book, *Lynda Madaras Talks to Teens About AIDS* (Newmarket Press, 1988). In fact, we urge all young people who are sexually active or are even thinking about having sex to read this book. It could literally save your life!

Other Health Issues: Pelvic Exams, Cervical Cancer, Precancerous Conditions of the Cervix, and Pap Smears

If you haven't yet begun having sexual intercourse, you don't really need to worry about these things yet. But, once you do, you will need to know about these diseases and to have regular pelvic exams and pap smears.

The girls in my classes usually have a lot of questions about these topics. Most of them have never even heard of precancerous conditions of the cervix before. This isn't very surprising; there are many adult women who don't know about this either. But it's very important, so we'd like you to read this section carefully. You might even ask your mom (or any adult woman you care about) to read this section, too, in case she doesn't know about these things.

What is a pelvic exam?

Pelvic exams, which are also called *gynecological* exams or *speculum* exams, are examinations of the female reproductive organs done by a doctor or nurse to make sure these organs are healthy. These exams may be done by a regular doctor, by a gynecologist (a doctor who specializes in female health care), or by a nurse practitioner who has special training in women's health care.

For the exam, you will first be asked to go to the bathroom in order to empty your bladder and then to undress and put on a gown or paper dress. First you may have your breasts examined in much the same way we described on pages 61–67 when we explained about breast self-exam. Next you will be asked to lie down on the exam table and to put your feet into the table's special stirrups. This can feel embarrassing because we're not used to being in this position or showing anyone these very private parts of our bodies. It might be less embarrassing for you if a woman does the exam. But, whether it's a woman or man, remember

pelvic (PEL-vick)
gynecological (GUY-neh-koh-LODGE-eh-cal)

that, even though it's new to you, the person has done this hundreds of times and is only interested in your health.

The doctor or nurse will then look at your vulva. Next, he or she may insert a lubricated, gloved finger into your vagina to gently push up on your uterus while using the other hand to press down on your abdomen. This is in order to feel the shape and outline of your uterus and ovaries. Sometimes the doctor or nurse may also insert a lubricated, gloved finger into your rectum in order to push your organs up higher.

After this, he or she will take a look inside your vagina using a speculum, an instrument that is inserted into the vagina and that pushes back the vaginal walls so the doctor or nurse can see inside. The insertion of the speculum and feeling inside your vagina with gloved fingers may feel a bit uncomfortable, especially if you are nervous or tense, but it shouldn't be painful. If it is painful, ask the doctor or nurse to stop. It may help you to feel more relaxed if you've had a chance to see your mom or someone else have a pelvic exam before you have your first one.

While the speculum is inside the vagina, the doctor or nurse may do a Pap smear (this test is discussed in more detail on pages 220–221). This involves gently rotating a small spatula or cotton swab around the cervix to collect some cells from its surface. You probably won't feel this very much. After this is done the speculum is removed. If you ask while the speculum is in, the doctor or nurse will give you a mirror so that you can look inside, too.

When should you have your first pelvic exam?
Some doctors say you should have your first pelvic exam once you've begun to menstruate. But as long as

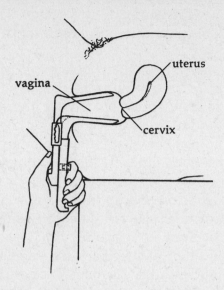

Illustration 44. The Speculum. Inserted in the vagina, the speculum pushes back the vaginal walls so the doctor or nurse can see inside.

you're healthy and don't have any problems with your menstrual cycle or any abnormal vaginal discharge that might be the sign of an infection, most doctors don't think you need to have an exam until you have begun having sexual intercourse. Once you've had your first exam, you should continue having one at least once a year.

What are cervical cancer and precancerous conditions of the cervix?
Cancer, as you may know, is a disease in which cells become so abnormal that they start to reproduce wildly, invade the surrounding tissue, spread to other parts of the body, and interfere with the body's normal, healthy functioning. Cervical cancer is a type of cancer that affects the cervix, the entrance to the uterus (see Illustration 21 on page 88).

Precancerous conditions of the cervix are abnormalities in the cells of the tissue of the cervix which, if left untreated, may eventually turn into cervical cancer. Doctors use a number of different terms when referring to precancerous conditions of the cervix. Depending upon how widespread the condition is and on the degree of abnormality in the cells, a doctor may use any of the following terms to describe the precancerous condition: dysplasia, cervical intraepithelial neoplasia (CIN), or carcinoma-in-situ.

What causes cervical cancer and precancerous conditions of the cervix?

Although the exact cause of these diseases is not definitely known, there is a good deal of scientific evidence which suggests that they may be caused by sexually transmitted viruses such as the ones that cause genital warts or herpes. For this reason, many doctors consider precancerous and cancerous conditions of the cervix to be sexually transmitted diseases.

Are some women more likely to get these diseases than other women?

Yes. For instance, women who have a history of herpes or genital warts are at higher risk, that is, are more likely to get these diseases. For some unknown reason, women who smoke are also at a higher risk. Since these diseases may be transmitted sexually, the greater the number of sexual partners a woman has, the greater her chance of getting these diseases. (However, this doesn't mean that a woman with one of these diseases has necessarily had a large number of partners.) Women

speculum (SPECK-you-lum)
dysplasia (dis-PLAY-shuh)
intraepithelial (IN-trah-ep-eh-THEAL-ee-al)
neoplasia (knee-oh-PLAY-shuh)
carcinoma (car-sih-NO-ma)
situ (SIGHT-you)

who start their sex lives during their teen years are also at higher risk. This may be due to the fact that the tissues of the cervix go through a stage of being very vulnerable to cancer-causing agents during the teenage years. (Here again, this doesn't mean that someone with cervical cancer has necessarily started her sex life during her teens.)

Of course, a woman may have all these risk factors and never get these diseases, while women who don't have these risk factors can develop these conditions.

How does a woman know if she has one of these diseases?
There usually aren't any symptoms to alert a woman to the fact that she has these diseases. The precancerous conditions usually don't produce much in the way of symptoms. Even with cervical cancer, there may not be any symptoms, at least not at first. Fortunately, though, a Pap smear can detect these diseases.

What is a Pap smear?
The Pap smear is a simple, painless test that can be done during a pelvic exam. The doctor or nurse collects some cells from your cervix, in the manner we described earlier. These cells are smeared on a slide and examined under a microscope to make sure they don't show any signs of a cancerous or precancerous condition. Usually, the slide is sent to a laboratory for the microscope examination and the doctor or nurse will call you if the test was not normal.

What happens if your Pap smear results aren't normal?
This depends on exactly what the Pap smear report says. In some cases, you will be asked to come back in a few months for another Pap smear. In other cases, the doctor may want to do other tests to confirm the results of the Pap smear.

If it turns out that you do have a precancerous condition, the problem can usually be treated fairly simply right in the doctor's office by cryosurgery, a method of destroying the affected cells by freezing. Luckily, precancerous conditions are 100% curable.

It's rare for young women to have an actual cancer of the cervix, but when they do, a surgical operation is usually necessary. In its early stages, cervical cancer is usually curable; however, in advanced cases, a cure may not be possible. Women still die from cervical cancer, but most of them could have been saved if they'd had regular Pap smears to detect the disease in its earlier, curable stages. This is why it's so important for women to have regular Pap smears.

When should I begin having Pap smears? How often should I have one?

You should have your first Pap smear test within two years of the time when you first have sexual intercourse. After you've had your first one, you should continue having one at least once every three years. Many doctors feel the test should be done once a year, and we agree.

If you have a history of herpes or genital warts, or if you've had a precancerous condition of the cervix in the past, you may need to have Pap smears even more often than once a year.

Sexual Crimes

When we talk about sexual intercourse in class, I often find questions about sexual crimes in the "Everything You Ever Wanted to Know" question box. So, we want to discuss this topic, in case you too have questions about these things.

Parents sometimes worry about bringing up the topic

of sexual crimes with their children because they don't want to scare them. Many parents want to protect their children from even hearing about such terrible things. This is understandable, but the fact of the matter is, sexual crimes do happen. We feel that the best way to protect children from sexual crimes is to make sure they know about these things and are prepared to handle the situation if they become victims of a sexual crime.

The three types of sexual crimes we'll be talking about here are rape, incest, and child molesting.

Rape
Rape means forcing someone to have sex against his or her will. It can happen to anyone—to young children, to adults, to people of any age. Most rape victims are females, and most rapists are males. Theoretically, it's possible for a woman to hold a gun to a man's head and force him to have intercourse with her, or for a woman to force a person (male or female) to have oral-genital sex with her, or something like this. It is also possible for a male to be raped by another male. By and large, though, rape cases involve a male raping a female.

If you are a victim of rape, the most important thing is to get help right away. Some rape victims are so upset by what's happened that they just want to go home and try to forget the whole thing. But a rape victim needs medical attention as soon as possible. Even if the victim doesn't seem to have any serious injuries, there could be internal injuries that need medical attention. The victim also needs to be tested to make sure that he or she hasn't gotten a sexually transmitted disease from the rape. If the victim is a woman, she needs a test to make sure she isn't pregnant and she may want to take the morning-after pill to prevent pregnancy. (These tests are one reason why a victim shouldn't bathe or shower before seeking medical attention). And, a rape victim should seek help because he or she will need support to recover emotionally as well as physically.

If you are a rape victim, there are a number of ways to go about getting help. You can go to a hospital emergency room or call the police, who will take you to the hospital. There are Rape Hotlines in most big towns and cities. You can find the number of the hotline closest to your home in your telephone directory or by calling the information operator.

Incest and Child Molesting

Incest involves one member of a family being sexual with another family member. It may include anything from touching, feeling, or kissing the sex organs to actual sexual intercourse. Of course, it isn't incest when a husband and wife do these things with each other. But when it happens between other family members, it's called incest.

Most victims of incest are girls who are victimized by their fathers, stepfathers, brothers, or some other male relative, although it is also possible for a girl to be victimized by a female relative. Boys can also be victims of incest. When incest happens to a boy, it may be either a female or a male relative who victimizes him. Incest can happen to very young children, even to babies, as well as to older children and teenagers.

Brothers and sisters often engage in some form of sex play as they're growing up, which may involve "playing doctor" or pretending to be "mommy and daddy." This kind of sex play between brothers and sisters is very common. It isn't always considered incest and it isn't necessarily a harmful thing. But being forced or pressured to have sexual contact with a brother or sister *is* incest, and it can be very harmful.

Incest isn't always a forced thing, like rape. Because of the older person's position in the family, he (or she) may be able to pressure the child into doing sexual things without actually having to use force. Most incest victims are so bewildered by what's going on that they simply don't know how to stop it or prevent it from happening again.

Child molesting, like incest, may involve anything from touching, feeling, or kissing the sex organs to actual sexual intercourse. (The word *molest* means to bother or to harm). But child molesting is different from incest because the person doing the molesting isn't a family member. It may be a complete stranger, a friend of the child's parents, or some other older person. Boys as well as girls may be victims of a child molester.

If you are a victim of incest or child molesting, the most important thing to do is to *tell someone*. This can be a difficult thing to do, particularly if you are an incest victim.

The logical people to tell are your parents. (Of course, in cases of incest by a parent, you need to tell the other parent). However, some parents have trouble believing their children at first. If, for whatever reason, your parents won't believe you, you might tell another relative—an aunt or uncle, a grandparent, an older sister or brother—whom you feel *will* believe you. Or you could tell another adult—a teacher or counselor at school, a friend's mother or father, your minister or priest, or any other adult you trust. You can also call the Child Abuse Hotline. The number is 800-422-4453. This number is toll-free, which means you don't have to pay for the call and it won't show up on your phone bill.

The people who answer the phones there are specially trained and they understand what you're going through. (Some of them have been victims of sexual crimes themselves.) You don't have to give your name, and what you say is entirely confidential, so don't hesitate to call.

Victims of incest or child molesting often find it hard to come forward and tell someone. Sometimes the person who committed the crime has made the victim promise to keep it a secret. But, there are some promises and some secrets a person needn't keep, and this is definitely one of them. Or, the victims may find it hard to tell someone because they think that what happened is somehow their fault, or that they're to blame because they didn't stop it from happening. But, this just isn't true. These crimes are *always* the fault of the older person. The victim is *never* to blame and is *never* at fault in any way. Some victims don't tell because they are afraid the person will harm them or get back at them for telling. But, the police or other authorities can make sure the victim is *fully protected*.

Incest victims sometimes hesitate to tell because incest is a crime, and it's possible that telling could get the person who has committed the crime into trouble with the police. Even though most victims hate what's been done to them, some of them still don't want to see a relative sent to jail. Although involving the police may seem like a horrifying idea, it will be better for everyone in the end and will protect any brothers or sisters who may also be suffering abuse. Besides, those who commit incest aren't always sent to jail. If possible the judge sends the person for some form of psychiatric treatment, while at the same time making sure that you are protected from further abuse.

Some incest victims don't tell because they're afraid that the family will break up, their parents will get divorced, or things will get worse than they are. But, if incest is going on, things are already about as bad as they could be. The victim and the other family members also need help in dealing with the situation. However, no one can get the help they need unless the victim has the courage to take the first step and tell someone.

Most victims of incest and child molesting feel a mixture of anger, embarrassment, and shame. This can also make it hard to come forward and tell someone. But you have a right to protect yourself from being touched in ways that don't feel right to you. So even though you may feel embarrassed, it's important to tell someone. It's really the best thing for everyone.

On a Lighter Note

When we went back and reread this chapter and the previous one, we were a little worried about how it sounded. All this talk about things like miscarriages, stillbirths, birth defects, AIDS and other sexually transmitted diseases, and sex crimes isn't exactly upbeat or cheery. Even though we think it's important to give our readers the kind of information that's in these chapters, we thought to ourselves, "Gee, kids who read this might feel like a ton of bricks just fell on their heads."

In other words, we were afraid that these chapters might make kids feel worried, upset, or depressed. Reading about so many negative things, one right after the other, can be a bit hard to take. We want to remind you that most women don't have miscarriages or stillbirths; most have completely trouble-free pregnancies and give birth to beautiful, healthy babies. And most people never have to face problems like rape, incest, child molesting, or AIDS. Although people can and do get sexually transmitted diseases, in most cases, they can be easily cured, especially when they're treated properly. So you shouldn't let the negative things in these chapters make you terribly worried. They're only a small part of the story.

On the whole, sex and reproduction are wonderful experiences. In fact, being sexual with someone you truly love is about the most wonderful, terrific, absolutely great feeling in the world. When you're thinking about the negative things in these chapters, then, be sure you also keep in mind the great joy and satisfaction that having children and being sexual can bring.

CHAPTER 11

Romantic and Sexual Feelings

If a girl is thirteen and she's had her period and all she ever thinks about is boys and sex, is this normal?

I think I might be sex-crazy or something. I mean, I'm always thinking about girls, fantasizing, and I masturbate a lot, like almost every day. Do you think I'm okay?

These questions came out of the "Everything You Ever Wanted to Know" question box. Questions like these often come up because, as we go through puberty, many of us experience stronger romantic and/or sexual feelings than ever before in our lives. For some of us this means spending time imagining a passionate romance with a special someone, or having sexual fantasies. For some it means having the urge to masturbate more often. For some it means getting interested in the opposite sex, having crushes, or having a boyfriend or girlfriend.

These romantic or sexual feelings can be very strong. At times, it may even seem as if romance and sex are all you can think about! Some young people get so wrapped up that it's a bit scary for them. If, like the boy and girl who asked the above questions, you've been worried about your strong romantic or sexual feelings, it helps to know that these feelings are perfectly normal and natural and that a lot of people your age are going through the same thing.

Besides questions like ones above, there are also questions like these:

> How come all the other girls think about boys and getting dates and stuff and I don't even want to go out or have boyfriends or anything?

> My friends are always talking about girls and sex and everything. But, I'm just not interested in girls in a romantic way yet. Do you think there's something wrong with me?

When boys and girls ask questions like these, I explain that although puberty is a time of strong sexual or romantic feelings for many young people, not everyone experiences these feelings. Some boys and girls are more involved in sports, school, music, a job, or some other aspect of their lives. Just as we each have our own personal timetable of development when it comes to the body changes of puberty, so we each have our own personal timetable when it comes to romance and sexual interests. If you've worried that there's something wrong with you because everyone else your age is madly in love or all wrapped up in the opposite sex and you aren't interested in such things, you can stop worrying. There's nothing wrong with you. Your personal timetable is just different from theirs.

The boys and girls in my classes are curious about

anything and everything having to do with sex, and they're especially curious about the kinds of romantic and sexual feelings that young people have when they're growing up. We've talked about fantasies and masturbation elsewhere in this book, and we'll mention these topics again in this chapter, particularly in the last section which deals with the difference between feeling private and feeling guilty about sexual matters.

But having fantasies and masturbating are basically private things that you do by yourself. In this chapter, we'll be talking more about your sexual and romantic feelings that involve other people. We'll be talking about romantic and sexual relationships and about things like crushes, dating, falling in love, kissing, necking, petting, and other topics that come up in our classes. Of course, there isn't room in this one chapter to fully cover these topics, but we hope we can answer at least some of your questions. Before we get started talking about romantic and sexual feelings and relationships, though, we'd like to say a couple of things about friendships.

"Just Friends"

You may be one of those kids who becomes interested in the opposite sex in a new way, develops crushes, begins having boyfriends or girlfriends, or even starts dating during your puberty years. Or you may not experience these things. Either way, you'll undoubtedly notice that boy-girl relationships s' t to change as puberty rolls around and that things are quite a bit different than when you were younger.

When we're small children no one makes much of a fuss over the fact that two kids of the opposite sex are friends. Occasionally, people will make cracks about "puppy love," but it's just not a big deal if a little boy and girl play together, are best friends, spend the night at each others' houses, and so forth. As puberty approaches, though, things change. Suddenly, it's no longer okay to spend the night at your best friend's house if your best friend happens to be someone of the opposite sex. The other kids at school or the adults around suddenly start assuming that you must be more than "just friends," that you "like" each other in a romantic, boyfriend/girlfriend sort of way.

At least, the kids in my classes often complain that it's harder to be "just friends" after you reach a certain age. Here's what one girl in my class had to say about this:

> I'm going to Paul's Halloween party on Saturday, and my brother keeps teasing me, "Oh, you like Paul, you're in love with Paul." Well, I do like Paul, but not like that. All of a sudden, you can't just be friends with a boy. It's got to be boyfriend or girlfriend, like you're all romantic with each other.

An eleven-year-old boy who'd been friends with a girl since they were little kids had this to say:

> I went over to Hilary's house to spend the night, and we were swimming in the pool. These girls who live next door came over and they were saying things like, "Oh, you're playing with a girl. Oh, you're staying overnight at a girl's house. Oh, that's weird. You must be gay."
>
> Donny, age 11

Many kids complain about this sort of teasing and about people automatically assuming that a friend of the opposite sex is more than "just a friend." So, in class, we talk about how to handle this problem. Here's some advice we've come up with together:

- Just ignore the teasing and rumors.
- Explain to people that you *are* "just friends."
- Talk to your friend about it so the teasing or rumors don't make you feel uncomfortable around each other or affect your friendship.
- Don't worry about it too much because, when you're older, opposite-sex friendships aren't such a big deal anymore.
- "Turn things around" and act like the people who are teasing you are the ones who are weird for not being able to be friends with someone of the opposite sex.
- Take a "so what" attitude. After all, who cares if they think you're madly in love with your friend?
- Tell them why you think it's fun or a good idea or whatever to be "just friends" and what you get out of being close friends with someone of the opposite sex.
- Realize they may be jealous because they'd really like to have an opposite-sex friendship.

We think that the above suggestions are pretty good ones. So, if you're having problems in this way, take some of this advice, and don't let "the romance thing" keep you from enjoying an opposite-sex friendship.

Crushes

Of course, sometimes we are interested in romance. In fact, many boys and girls develop crushes. Having a crush means having romantic or sexual feelings towards a certain, special someone. Crushes can be very exciting. Just thinking about or catching a glimpse of the person you have a crush on can brighten your whole day, and you may spend delightful hours imagining a romance with him or her.

Sometimes boys and girls develop crushes on someone who isn't very likely to return their affections—a film star, a rock singer, a teacher or other adult, or a friend of an older brother or sister. These sorts of crushes can be a safe and healthy way of experimenting with romantic and sexual attractions—no matter how much we may pretend otherwise, deep down we know that this person is unattainable. So, we don't have to worry about real-life problems like what to say or how to act. We're free to imagine what we like, without worrying about whether that person will be attracted to us. In a way, having a crush on someone unattainable is a way of rehearsing for the time in our lives when we will have a real-life romance.

But having a crush on someone unattainable can also cause a lot of suffering. One year some of the girls in my class developed crushes on a certain rock star. They plastered their bedroom walls with posters, wore buttons with his face printed on them, pored over fan magazines, and generally had a great time sharing their feelings about him with one another. When the rock star got married, they were, naturally, somewhat disappointed, but one girl was more than disappointed. She was really upset. She had gotten too involved in her crush, and the rock star's marriage was devastating for her. If you find yourself developing a serious crush on someone unattainable, it helps to remind yourself from time to time that your crush isn't very realistic and that this person isn't very likely to return your affections.

Not all crushes are unrealistic. You may develop a crush on someone near your own age whom you actually know through school, church, temple, or some other group. If that person shows an interest in you as well, the crush can be especially exciting. But yearning after a person who doesn't return your affections can be painful. If you find that your crushes are causing you problems, it helps to find someone—a friend, a parent, a teacher, another adult, or a counselor—with whom you can discuss your feelings.

When we talk about crushes and being romantically or sexually interested in a certain, special someone you've actually met or know, I'm often asked questions like these:

How do you find out if someone likes you? How do you let someone know you like them?
There are basically two ways: You can do it on your own, or you can have a friend do it for you.

If you decide to have a friend do it, you'll want to pick someone you really trust, or next thing you know it will be all over school! It's often easier to let someone else do the talking for you. But keep in mind that, if you do this, you don't have very much control over what's being said. Suppose, for example, you only want your friend to bring up your name in a roundabout way and see how this other person reacts. Instead, your friend might tell this other person that you're madly in love with him or her!

For these reasons, many people prefer doing it on their own. You can let someone know you like him or her by being friendly, starting conversations, going out of your way to be around that person, asking the person to go out with you, or simply telling the person how you feel. You can also find out if a person likes you by watching to see if that person does any of these sorts of things to *you*.

Regardless of whether you tell the person yourself or have a friend do it for you, make sure it's done in private and not in front of your other friends or classmates. Otherwise, the person may be so embarrassed that he or she may say they don't like you even if they really do!

Dating

As young people move through puberty and into their teen years, many begin dating. This can be fun and exciting, but it can also create problems. For instance, you may want to date before your parents think you're old enough. Or you may not feel ready to date, and your parents or friends may be pushing you into it. You may have trouble deciding whether you want to go steady with one person or go out with lots of different people. If you've been dating one person regularly and decide you want to date others, you may have problems in ending your steady dating relationship. Or, if your steady boyfriend or girlfriend decides to change the relationship, you may have a hard time coping with this. On the other hand, if you want to date and no one is interested in going out with you, you may feel rather depressed.

Here again, if you're having problems that relate to dating, it might be helpful for you to talk them over with someone you respect and trust. One of your parents, another adult you trust, a friend, or an older brother or sister might be someone you could talk to. You might also want to take a look at our book, *Lynda Madaras' Growing Up Guide for Girls* (Newmarket Press, 1986), which talks about these issues. Even though this book was written for girls, lots of boys have found it useful, too. In addition, it might be helpful for you to hear some of the questions that come up in my classes about this topic.

Suppose that you'd like to date, but you never have and you're beginning to wonder if you ever will?
If the other kids you know have already started dating, but you haven't, you may get to feeling that these things won't ever happen to you. If so, it helps to

remember that, just as we each have our own special timetable of development when it comes to the physical changes of puberty, so we each have our own time-tables when it comes to romantic matters. It can be awfully hard if your personal timetable is moving along more slowly than other people's. But the fact that you're getting a slow start doesn't mean that you won't ever start dating. It may take a while, but eventually, you'll start dating too. We guarantee it!

Remember, you've got many years ahead of you. It doesn't really matter if you start dating when you're only twelve years old or not until you're twenty. What's important in the long run is that you feel good about yourself.

Is it all right for a girl to ask a boy out?
We think so. Although there are still some people who think it's not "right" or "proper" for girls to do the asking, most people don't see anything at all wrong with a girl taking the initiative. In fact, many people think it's a great idea. Almost every boy we've ever asked has said he wished more girls would do it. Girls are often in favor of this idea, too. However, many girls have admitted to being so worried about what others might think, or so afraid that the boy might say "no," that they can't bring themselves to actually ask a boy out.

Our opinion: *Go for it!* After all, the worst that could happen is that you'll be turned down, and that wouldn't really be the end of the world. Besides, if a girl waits to be asked, she may never be asked. As one girl put it, "My boyfriend is so shy. We'd never have gotten together if I hadn't gotten the ball rolling by asking him out. I'm glad I did!"

What if every time you ask someone out, the answer is "no"?

If you've asked a boy out a number of times and he keeps saying "no," then you may just have to face the fact that he doesn't want to go out with you. It can be difficult to know exactly how many times you should ask before giving up altogether. Partly, it will depend on what he says when turning you down. If he tells you that he's already dating someone else or simply isn't interested in you, then that's a pretty clear sign that you should stop asking. But, if he says, "I'm sorry, but I'm busy," or doesn't give a clear reason for saying "no," you might want to try again. Perhaps he really is busy, but would like to go out with you another time. But if you've tried a few times and have gotten this kind of reply, you might want to say something like, "Is there a time when we could get together?" The answer to this question will usually give you a clear idea of whether it's worth your while to keep asking this person out.

If you've asked a number of different boys out and all of them have said "no," you may begin feeling awfully discouraged. You may even start to feel that there's something so wrong or so horrible about you that no one will ever say "yes." But, before you allow yourself to feel down and discouraged, think for a moment about who you're asking out—maybe they're the wrong people! Are you only asking the best-looking or most popular boys? If so, this may be part of your problem. For one thing, the best-looking and most popular boys may already have lots of people asking them out, so your chances aren't as good as if you asked someone less popular or not-totally-gorgeous. Besides, the fact that someone is popular or good-looking doesn't necessarily mean you're going to have a great time with him. What's more important is whether he's nice, whether the two of you could be comfortable with each other, whether you could have fun together. The person's inner qualities are a lot more important than other qualities like being popular or good-looking.

You might also ask yourself how well you know the person you're asking out. If you're asking someone you hardly know, this may be a big part of the reason you keep getting turned down. If you take the time to get to know someone and to let him get to know you first, you'll have a better chance of having him say "yes" when you ask for a date.

It might also be helpful for you to have a mutual friend check things out before you ask for a date. Your friend can give you an idea of how he might respond. If he isn't interested, you'll save yourself the discouragement of being turned down again. In addition, you might ask some of your friends who they think you should ask for a date. People love to play matchmaker, and your friends may come up with someone you wouldn't have thought of on your own. They may even know someone who's been dying to go out with you! So don't hesitate to enlist your friends' help.

Suppose you want to date, but your parents say "no"?
Young people usually choose to handle this problem in one of three ways: 1) Sneak around behind their parents' backs; 2) Go along with their parents' rules and wait until their parents say they're old enough; 3) Try and change their parents' minds. Let's look at each of these choices.

Sneaking around just isn't a good idea. If you get caught, you may get into a lot of trouble, and your parents may find it hard to trust you in the future. Even if you don't get caught, you'll probably feel awfully guilty about lying, which isn't much fun.

On the other hand, it can be awfully hard to go along with your parents' rules and wait until you're older, especially if there's a special someone you'd like to date. But parents usually aren't trying to be mean or unfair. They're trying to protect you from "getting in over your head" by dating at too young an age. Maybe they're right. If your parents say "no," ask yourself these questions: Are the other kids my age allowed to go out? Would I really lose anything by waiting until I'm older?

If your honest answer to these two questions is "no," then perhaps waiting is the best choice for you. If, however, you feel that your parents are being too strict or too old-fashioned, you might want to consider the third choice, changing their minds.

This may not be easy, but it's worth a try. For starters, find out exactly why they've made these rules. What are they worried about? Once you hear them out, you may be able to come up with a compromise. If, for instance, your parents think you're too young to go out on a solo date, maybe they'd allow you to go on group dates. Or, if they won't allow dates for the movies, perhaps they'll allow you to go to a boy–girl party or invite someone to your house.

How do you know if it's really love?
Once they begin dating, many young people fall in love, or at least what they think might be love, so they ask questions like the one above.

Emotions can't be weighed or measured and different people have different ideas of what it means to be in love. So, we can't give you a definite answer to this question. But we can share with you some of our thoughts on the subject.

We think it's important to recognize the differences between infatuation and true love. *Infatuation* is an intense, exciting (and sometimes confusing or scary) fireworks kind of feeling. You may be so wrapped up in your infatuation that it's hard to think about anything else. People sometimes mistake infatuation for love. But infatuation usually doesn't last very long; true love does. You may start out being infatuated and have it grow into true love. Or, the infatuation may pass and you may discover that you weren't really "right" for each other, after all. In addition, you don't have to know someone very well in order to be infatuated. But in order to truly love someone, you have to know that person (both their good qualities and bad ones) very well. In addition, infatuation can happen all of a sudden. True love takes more time.

Regardless of whether your relationship starts with the fireworks, infatuation-kind-of-feeling or develops more slowly and gradually, sooner or later love relationships go through a questioning stage, where one or both of you begin to question whether this relationship is really a good one. During this questioning stage, one or the other of you may decide to end the relationship. In our opinion, it's only after you go through this questioning stage and decide to stay together that you're really on the road to true love.

Homosexual Feelings

This is another topic that always comes up when we talk in class about the sexual and romantic feelings people have during their growing-up years. *Homo* means "same." Having *homosexual feelings* means having romantic or sexual thoughts, fantasies, dreams, attractions, or crushes that involve someone who is the same sex as we are. Many boys and girls have homosexual thoughts or feelings, or actual sexual experiences with someone of the same sex, while they're growing up.

If you've had homosexual feelings or experiences, you may realize that this is quite normal, and you may not be at all worried about it. Or, you may feel somewhat confused or upset, or even downright scared, about having these kinds of feelings or experiences. Perhaps you've heard people making jokes or using insulting slang terms when talking about homosexuality. If so, this may have caused you to wonder if your homosexual feelings or experiences are really okay. Perhaps you have heard someone say that homosexuality is morally wrong, sinful, abnormal, or a sign of mental sickness. If so, this, too, may have made you wonder or worry about your own feelings. If you've heard any of these things (or even if you haven't), we think it will be helpful for you to know the basic facts about homosexuality.

Although almost everyone has homosexual feelings or experiences at some time or another in their lives, we usually consider people to be homosexuals only if, as adults, their strongest romantic and sexual attractions are towards someone of the same sex, or most of their actual sexual experiences involve someone of the same sex.

Both males and females may be homosexuals. Female homosexuals are also called *lesbians*. "Gay" is a non-insulting slang term for both male and female homosexuals. There have been homosexuals throughout history—some very famous. People from any social class, ethnic background, religious affiliation, or economic level may be homosexual. Doctors, nurses, lawyers, bus drivers, police officers, artists, business people, ministers, rabbis, priests, teachers, politicians, football play-

lesbians (LES-be-anz)

ers, married people, single people, parents: you name it—all sorts of people are homosexuals.

The majority of adults in our society are *heterosexual* people (hetero means "opposite") whose strong romantic and sexual attractions are towards the opposite sex and whose actual sexual experiences mostly involve the opposite sex. However, about one in every ten adults is a homosexual. Although an adult is usually considered either a homosexual or a heterosexual, this doesn't mean that he or she doesn't sometimes have feelings or experiences in the other direction. Very few people are *strictly* homosexual or *strictly* heterosexual.

Now that you know a bit about homosexuality, you might want to read some questions that the students in my classes have asked and the answers to these questions.

Is homosexuality morally wrong? Is it unnatural, abnormal, or a sign of a mental sickness?
In the past, many people felt that homosexuality was sinful or abnormal, and there are still some people who think it's morally wrong or a sign of mental illness that needs to be cured by a psychiatrist. However, nowadays, many people no longer believe this. They feel that it's a personal matter, that some people just happen to be homosexuals, and that being homosexual is a perfectly healthy, normal, and acceptable way to be.

What's a bisexual?
A bisexual is a person who is equally attracted to males and females and whose sexual activities may involve either sex.

If a person has a lot of homosexual feelings or fools around with someone of the same sex while growing up, will this person be a homosexual as an adult?
Having homosexual feelings and experiences while you're growing up has *nothing at all* to do with whether

or not you'll be homosexual as an adult. Some of the young people who have homosexual feelings and experiences while they're growing up turn out to be homosexuals as adults and some turn out to be heterosexuals. Some adult homosexuals had homosexual feelings while they were growing up; others had heterosexual feelings; still others didn't have strong feelings one way or the other as they were growing up.

Can a person know for sure that they're gay even though they're still young?
Yes. At least, some gay adults say that they knew they were homosexuals when they were teens, or even when they were very small children.

How can I find out more about homosexuality?
If you would like more information about homosexuality, you might be interested in some of the books listed at the back of this book on pages 260-263. You can also contact the Gay and Lesbian Community Service Center, 1213 North Highland Avenue, Los Angeles, CA 90038. They publish a newsletter called REACH, which is written for and by gay teens, and they will send you a free copy in a plain envelope if you request it. In addition, their Temenos Youth Outreach program sponsors a pen pal program, and on Fridays and Saturdays from 7:00 p.m. to midnight, West Coast time, they have a talk line for gay teens (213-462-8130).

Is there anything else I should know about homosexuality?
Yes. You should know that male homosexuals and male bisexuals are at higher risk of getting AIDS, a deadly sexually transmitted disease that is passed through contact with infected body fluids such as blood, semen, urine, or feces. Homosexual activity that involves the exchange of these body fluids could lead to AIDS if one or the other person has the AIDS virus in his or her

244 Romantic and Sexual Feelings

body. So, males who have sexual contact with homosexuals or bisexuals should pay special attention to the section on AIDS on pages 202-215 of this book. The Gay and Lesbian Health Center listed also has a free pamphlet and information on "safe sex."

Making Decisions About How to Handle Your Romantic and Sexual Feelings

Once young people begin going out, they often find themselves faced with questions about how to handle the strong romantic and sexual feelings they may be having. When two people are attracted to each other, they quite naturally want to be physically close. Being physically close may mean something as simple as holding hands or kissing goodnight after a date. Or, it may mean more than this. Physical closeness may even include something as intimate as sexual intercourse.

Some young people don't have much trouble in deciding what kind of physical closeness is right for them or in making decisions about "how far" they want to go in terms of physical intimacy. Such young people have strong moral or religious beliefs or other values that guide them in making these sorts of decisions. But other young people aren't sure what's right or wrong when it comes to deciding how far to go. And even those who *are* sure sometimes have a difficult time sticking to their beliefs once they're actually in a romantic situation. So, I usually spend a good deal of time, especially in my classes for older boys and girls, discussing the topic of making decisions about how to handle romantic and sexual feelings. There isn't enough space here to cover everything we discuss in class, but in the following pages we'll answer some of the most frequently asked questions.

If there were one set of answers that everyone agreed with, it would be easy to answer these sorts of questions, and our job as sex education teacher/writers would be much easier. But, it's not that simple: Different people have different ideas on these issues, and many of them feel quite strongly about their point of view. So we try to present these many different opinions as thoroughly as possible, and explain why people feel the way they do, without "taking sides" one way or the other. We think it's important for young people to hear all sides of a question and come up with their own answers, rather than just going along with someone else's opinion. For example, some young people answer questions about how to handle their sexual and romantic feelings based on what they think "everyone else" is doing. Not only are they often wrong about what "everyone else" is doing, but the fact of the matter is that *just because "everyone else" does it, does not mean it's right for you.*

Or, to take another example, some young people don't think through these issues on their own and just "go along" with what their parents or their religions say is right or wrong. Now, please don't misunderstand what we're saying here. We're not saying that you shouldn't follow your parents' or your religion's teachings or rules. In fact, we think parents and religions have excellent advice that's well worth following. But we've found that young people who just accept what they've been taught without thinking things through for themselves frequently run into problems when they're actually in situations where they have to make decisions about "how far" to go. Oftentimes, they aren't able to stick to the rules they've been taught. The rules sort of "fall apart" or "cave in" in the face of the tremendous pressure to experiment sexually that's often put on young people. We think this happens because the rules weren't really "theirs" in the first place; they come from someone else. Not until you consider all the different viewpoints and decide for yourself what rules to follow will the rules become truly your own. And it's not until the rules are truly your own that they become rules you can live by.

I'd like to have a boyfriend, but is someone my age (eleven) old enough to have sex? I'm twelve and there's a certain boy in my class that I like, and he likes me, too. I'm scared of having sex, though. What should I do? We kissed goodnight after our first date. I want to go out with him again, but what if I get pregnant?

It's usually younger boys and girls who ask these sorts of questions. When I first heard questions like these, I was a bit shocked that boys and girls who were so young seemed to be asking questions about whether they were ready for sex. However, in talking further with the young kids who asked these sorts of questions, I realized that the reason they were asking these questions was often because they had very mistaken ideas about physical intimacy. Some of them thought that kissing or being physically close in other ways happens almost as soon as you get involved with someone, or at least very quickly—perhaps even before you've had a chance to get to know each other. Some thought that going on a date means you have to, at the very least, kiss the person goodnight or perhaps even go further. Some even thought that having a boyfriend or girlfriend automatically means that you're going to have sexual intercourse with that person.

These things just aren't true, but it's easy to see how kids get these mistaken ideas. In the books we read, it often seems as if two people who meet on one page will be madly kissing each other on the next page. In the movies, it sometimes seems as if two perfect strangers take one look at each other, and the next thing we know they're in bed together!

But in real life, things don't usually happen quite like this. A romantic relationship usually goes through several steps or stages of physical closeness before sexual intercourse occurs, if indeed the relationship ever goes that far.

So please don't be confused by what you read in books or see on TV or in the movies. Dating or having boyfriends doesn't mean that you have to have sex or kiss or even just hold hands. Above all, remember that when it comes to romance and sex, you're in charge and you don't have to do anything that doesn't feel right for you.

What is French-kissing? What's the right way to French-kiss?
French-kissing, which some people call tongue-kissing, means that one or both people put their tongues in the other person's mouth while kissing. Some people like French-kissing; other don't and choose not to do it. There is no "right" or "wrong" way to French-kiss. Some people just put the tip of their tongue into the other person's mouth. Others put more of their tongue in; still others manage to get their tongues in each other's mouth at the same time. There just aren't any specific rules about this.

What is necking? What is petting?
Necking—or "making out" as some people call it— means having prolonged kissing sessions. Different people define "petting" differently. Some people use the phrase "petting above the waist" or "light petting" to describe a situation in which a male feels or fondles a female's breasts. "Petting below the waist" or "heavy petting" means touching or rubbing the other person's

genital organs. Some people further divide petting into "petting outside or over your clothes" and "petting inside or under your clothes."

What is mutual masturbation? What do people mean when they say "doing everything but"? What does "going all the way" mean?
Mutual masturbation means masturbating while another person also masturbates, or masturbating each other. "Doing everything but" means that although two people stop short of actually having sexual intercourse, they engage in other forms of physical closeness such as heavy petting; getting naked or partially naked and hugging, rubbing, or touching each other's bodies; mutual masturbation; oral-genital sex; or other intimate sexual contact. "Going all the way" means having sexual intercourse, that is, the male putting his penis in the female's vagina.

Is it all right to kiss on your first date? Is it wrong to get into necking? How about petting? How far is "too far" to go? Where should you draw the line? Is it okay to "do everything but," as long as you don't "go all the way" and have sex?
As we explained earlier, if everyone agreed upon these issues, these would be easy questions to answer. But, of course, they don't. For instance, some people think it's not right to kiss on a first date, while others think it's perfectly okay to do so. Some people think necking is okay; others don't. Some people think it's "sinful" to go beyond necking or, perhaps, light petting. Some don't think this is morally wrong, but are afraid that young people might get "too carried away" or "too turned on" and wind up going further than they really meant to. Other people have still other opinions on these issues, and some people just aren't certain exactly *how* to answer these sorts of questions.

Young people's answers to the sorts of questions listed above are strongly influenced by their personal situations—by their parents' values, their friend's opinions, their religion's teachings, their own moral beliefs, and their own emotional feelings. These influences affect each of us differently, but we think there are some basic guidelines that are helpful to anyone facing these questions, regardless of their personal situation, morals, or values:

1. Whether it's French-kissing, petting, or going further, don't let yourself be rushed into anything. Do only what you're really sure you want to do. After all, you have many years ahead of you; you can afford to wait until you are sure.
2. Ask yourself how you feel about this other person. Is this someone you trust? Will this person start rumors or gossip about you? Are you doing these things because you really care about this person or simply because you're curious to try these things? Young people are naturally curious about how it feels to neck, pet, or do some of these other things, but remember that it may not be as pleasurable if you're only doing it out of curiosity.
3. Ask yourself *why* you want to do this. Your real reasons may not have much to do with your feelings about the other person or even with your curiosity about these things. You may actually be hoping to prove you're grown up, trying to become more popular, or afraid you'll "lose" him or her if you don't. But agreeing to kiss, neck, pet, or go further for these reasons doesn't solve any of these problems. In fact, it may create new ones.
4. Don't pressure someone into doing something he or she doesn't want to do. This pressure may take the form of a boy persuading a girl to go further than she really wants to, or of a girl acting like a boy isn't "manly" if he doesn't want to kiss or doesn't try to get her to go further.
5. Don't allow yourself to fall for a "line," such as: "If you liked me, you'd neck with me"; "If you truly cared about me, you wouldn't say no"; "If you don't, I'll find someone else who will"; "Everybody else is doing it." If someone hands you one of these lines, turn the line back on them: "If you truly cared about me, you wouldn't pressure me"; "Prove you love me by not pushing me"; "So go ahead and

find someone else"; "If everybody else is doing it, you shouldn't have much trouble finding someone to do it with you."

6. Don't assume you know what the other person is thinking— *ask*. Many boys and girls get involved in necking, petting, or other sexual activities even though they don't really want to, just because they think the other person wants or expects to do these things. But this isn't always the case. Sometimes neither of you really wants to, so talk things over first.

7. Don't be afraid to say "no." Sometimes young people get involved in doing something because they're afraid they'll hurt someone's feeings if they refuse. We're all taught not to be selfish or hurt another's feelings. But your sexuality is one aspect of your life you have a right to be selfish about, so if you don't want to, it's okay to say "no."

8. Don't be too hard on yourself if you make a mistake and afterwards find that you've done something you wished you hadn't. Learning to make decisions about how to handle your romantic and sexual feelings is just like learning anything else: you're bound to make mistakes. Remember, too, that if you have done something you regret, you can always decide to behave differently in the future.

How old should you be before you start having sex? Should you wait until you're married? Is it okay to have sex if you're really in love, even though you're not married? Are teenagers mature enough to handle sex? Why do people make such a big fuss about sex? I mean, if two people want to have sex, why shouldn't they just go ahead and do it?

Even though each of these questions is phrased a bit differently, they are all about the same thing—when is it all right for a person to have sex and when isn't it? Once again, there isn't just one set of agreed-upon rules, and different people have different ideas on this subject.

Some people feel it's acceptable for two people to have sex with each other as long as they're both adults or have reached a certain age. Some of these people consider a person to be an adult once he or she has reached a specific age, such as eighteen or twenty-one.

Others think you're an adult once you're out on your own, that is, once you're no longer living with your parents and/or you're earning your own living and supporting yourself. Still others have what we call the "legal" point of view. They feel it's all right for people to have sex as long as they're over the legal age limit, which varies from state to state.

However, for most people, it's not *how old* you are that's the important thing. For instance, many people feel that you shouldn't have sex until you're married, regardless of your age. People who have the "wait until you're married" point of view may have this opinion for a variety of different reasons. For some, it's religious. They feel that the Bible tells us very clearly that people should not have sex unless they're married to each other. Others are concerned about what will happen if an unmarried couple has sex and a pregnancy results. Such people are often morally opposed to abortion. They feel that a decision to have sex isn't just a decision between two people but a choice that involves the responsibility for a third person, the baby that might be conceived. For this reason, they feel that you shouldn't have sex until you're married and are able to take on the responsibility of raising a child.

There are also other reasons why people have a "wait until you're married" point of view. One man we interviewed, whom we'll call Charlie, explained his reasons particularly well. Charlie was not a religious person, but as he explains, he decided not to have sex until he was married:

> My wife and I waited until we were married to have sex, which is unusual nowadays. But I think it was a good decision. Maybe if we'd had sex with other people or with each other before we were married, we'd have been more experienced or knowledgeable. But learning about sex together made it that much more special. We didn't have to

worry if either of us was as good as the other lovers either of us might have had before.

By being willing to wait until we were married, I felt I was showing my wife that it wasn't just sex that I wanted from her but real, true love and a lifelong commitment. And she was showing me the same thing. We really trusted each other, and that made us feel safe enough to really let go. We didn't have to worry that if we did it wrong or it wasn't great the first time that it would be all over. And, in fact, it wasn't so great the first time. It was kind of awkward and embarrassing. But I knew and she knew that we'd both be around tomorrow. This trust and commitment made us able to grow to be better lovers than we might otherwise have been.

While some people feel strongly about waiting until you're married or until you've reached a certain age, others put more emphasis on maturity or on the nature of the relationship. For instance, some people feel it's all right to have sex if you're really in love. Some say it's all right even if you're not in love, as long you're really committed to a serious, long-term relationship. Some say it's all right as long as you're both mature enough to handle it.

Of course, it's not always easy to know for sure if it's really love, just how serious or long-lasting the relationship will be, or whether you're really mature enough to handle it. But people who have these kinds of guidelines are concerned about the emotional feelings involved in sex. Having sexual intercourse involves very intense emotional feelings, and it's very easy for people to be hurt. When parents don't want teenagers to have sex, many times they're concerned not only about morality or the possibility of pregnancy, but also about the emotional pain that can result when the relationship ends. Also, as Charlie pointed out, sex is something that takes some time to work out. If two people aren't in love or in a long-term relationship that guarantees that the other person will be around to work things out with, one or both people may suffer emotionally.

One young woman we interviewed had something especially interesting to say about why she thought it was important to wait to have sex until you were involved in a serious relationship:

> I have girlfriends who think if you get into heavy petting and all that with a boy, it's stupid or artificial or something not to go all the way and have sex with him. They say sex isn't such a big deal. Maybe I'm too romantic or too idealistic, but I think sex *is* a big deal, or should be. I want it to be very deep and very emotional. . . . I know you can go around having sex all the time and it *won't* be a big deal for you. If you do that too much, though, I think you get, well, hard and cold and kind of callous. It's like you deaden yourself: you're no longer even capable of having it be deep or emotional.

There are also some people who don't place much importance on being in love or in a serious relationship. These people feel that if two people are attracted to each other and want to have sex, then it's perfectly acceptable for them to do so. Such people often feel that society is "too uptight" or "too hung up" about sex. They argue that sex is normal and natural and that people should be free to enjoy it whenever they want to, provided, of course, that both people consent to do so. Some people even go so far as to say that it's all right for two people to have sex even if they've just met or hardly know each other. However, not everyone who approves of casual sex is quite this casual about it.

As we've explained, there are many moral, religious, and emotional reasons why people don't feel that casual sex is a wise idea. There are also health reasons. Having casual sex increases your chances of getting sexually transmitted diseases (STDs). STDs can have serious, and in the case of AIDS, even deadly, consequences. Because of these health issues, many people today feel that casual sex is just far too risky.

So far, we've talked about people who have one certain viewpoint or another, but there are also many people who simply aren't sure how they feel about the question of when it's all right for people to have sex. If you're one of these, you might find it useful to talk this over with other people. In the end, only you can answer these questions and make your own decisions about how to handle your sexuality.

Don't (as many young people do) automatically rule out your parents as people to talk to. You may be surprised to find that your parents struggled with these same questions when they were your age. Young people often don't talk about sexual decision-making with their parents because they already know that their parents' attitudes are more conservative or stricter than theirs. But even if this is so, your parents may have good reasons for feeling the way they do. And even if you don't totally agree with them, they might have things to say that could prove useful to you. You might also talk with other people, an aunt or uncle, a sister or brother, or an older friend.

Sexuality: Feeling Private/Feeling Guilty

Even though we haven't actually used the word *sexuality*, we've been talking about sexuality throughout this chapter—and in fact, throughout this whole book. Some people think the word sexuality only applies to sexual intercourse, but it also includes such things as your general attitudes about sex, feelings about your changing body, romantic and sexual fantasies, masturbation, childhood sex play, homosexual feelings, crushes, hugging, kissing, petting, and being physically close in other ways.

Feeling Private

Most people feel private, shy, or even a bit embarrassed about some aspect of their sexuality. Some young people, for instance, become very modest during puberty, and no longer feel okay about family members seeing them nude. Some feel embarrassed asking questions or talking about the changes happening in their bodies. Some feel very private about starting their periods or having wet dreams and don't want their families or friends to know that these things have happened.

Private feelings can also center around romantic and sexual feelings or activities. Some kids are shy about the fact that they have a crush. Others feel embarrassed about their fantasies or about homosexual feelings. For most, masturbation is something that's very private. Young people may also feel shy about things like kissing, necking, petting, and other kinds of physical closeness. Some feel embarrassed even talking about these things, let alone actually doing them.

Some kids even worry about the fact that sexuality is such a private thing for them. But, feeling private, shy, or even a bit embarrassed about sexuality is completely natural. It doesn't mean that you're "hung up" or "uptight" or that there's something wrong with you. It just means that you're normal!

Feeling Guilty

There is, however, a difference between feeling *private* about your sexuality and feeling *guilty* about it. Some kids don't just feel private, shy, or embarrassed, they also feel guilty, ashamed, "dirty," or otherwise bad about some aspect of their sexuality.

When young people tell us they're having these guilty feelings, we suggest that they ask themselves if what they're feeling guilty about is something that is (or could be) harmful to themselves or others. If it's not, then our advice is to try and let go of the guilty feelings. If, on the other hand, it is something that's harmful, our advice is to make amends (if possible), to stop doing whatever it is that has caused the guilty feelings, and to decide not to do it in the future.

Even when a person *has* done something harmful, it's often something that's not too serious. For instance, you might feel guilty if you'd been flirting with your best friend's steady. But this isn't really all that serious. At least, it's not as serious as the kind of situation described by a fifteen-year-old boy who was feeling guilty about having pressured his girlfriend to go further than she really wanted to:

> Necking is as far as she'd ever go because of her moral standards. I kept pushing and got her to, well . . . not actual intercourse, but further than she wanted to go. I didn't force her or anything. I was coming on strong, though. Now I feel like some kind of pervert, and I can tell she doesn't feel good about herself. It's changed things between us. We're not so close.

This boy had done something that was harmful to his girlfriend's good feelings about herself and to his own good feelings about himself. It also hurt their relationship.

In other cases, the harm may be even more serious.

sexuality (SEK-shoo-AL-eh-tee)

If, for example, you didn't tell a sex partner that you had a sexually transmitted disease, or if an unwanted pregnancy resulted from the fact that you didn't use contraception, then the harm done could be quite serious indeed. Generally speaking, the more serious the harm, the harder it is to deal with the guilt. And, even though you've changed your behavior and done what you can to make amends, this doesn't mean your guilt will go away completely.

It's important to remember that human beings are, after all, *human*. We do make mistakes. If you've done what you can to make amends and change your behavior, then it's important to forgive yourself and get on with your life.

We also want to remind you of the fact that different people have different ideas about what is or isn't harmful. Take, for example, masturbation, which is something many young people feel guilty about. Personally we think masturbating is a perfectly normal, perfectly healthy thing to do. Unless it goes against a person's moral principles (in which case it could be a harmful thing for that particular person), we usually advise young people who are feeling guilty about masturbating to try and relax and let go of the guilt. However, some people see things quite differently. They believe that masturbation is sinful or morally wrong and that people do themselves harm in a moral sense by masturbating. Because of these beliefs their advice would probably be just the opposite of ours. They might advise young people to stop masturbating, and to decide not to masturbate again in the future.

How people react to situations where they feel guilty will depend, then, not only on how serious any harm done may be, but also on their ideas as to what is or isn't harmful. It's also possible for young people to feel guilty about doing something that few people, if any, would consider harmful at all. For instance, one sixteen-year-old girl who wrote to us said:

> If I just kiss a boy goodnight I feel so ashamed, not while I'm kissing but afterwards. I know it's not normal to feel so guilty, yet I do. How can I get over feeling so guilty?

This girl felt guilty and ashamed simply for kissing a boy good-night. And, judging from the letters we get, she's not alone. Some kids feel guilty even though they haven't actually *done* anything at all. For example, some boys and girls have told us that they felt not just shy or embarrassed, but also ashamed, of the fact that they've gotten their periods or had wet dreams.

Kids who feel this ashamed—or, for that matter, any young people who are feeling guilty about their sexuality even though they haven't done anything harmful—may find it helpful to think about *why* they feel this way. Often it's because some important person (often a parent) or group (maybe a religion, a government, or just society in general) has taught or influenced them to feel this way. Until fairly recently in our history, most people in our society had *very* negative attitudes about sexuality. In your great grandparents' day, sexual thoughts and feelings were often considered evil, the work of the devil. Sexual desires were considered impure or unclean, especially in women. Women who felt sexual urges or who enjoyed sex were considered abnormal, sick, or perverted. Many people felt it was sinful even for married people to have sex, unless they were trying to have a child.

Of course, times change and so do people's attitudes. Today, most people in our society have more positive attitudes about sexuality, but there are still many people who have very negative, or at least somewhat negative, attitudes about sexuality. Parents who have these attitudes may pass them on to their children. Even though parents may not actually come out and say "sexuality is bad," they may pass these attitudes on in other ways. A parent might, for instance, get upset when a little baby touches his or her sex organs and move the baby's hand away or even slap them. This may give the baby the idea that sex organs are "nasty" or "dirty" and that it's "wrong" or "bad" to touch them. Thus, when that baby grows up, he or she may feel ashamed about menstruation or wet dreams or may feel guilty about masturbating.

When you think about it this way, it's really not surprising that some kids feel guilty about sexuality even though they haven't actually done anything that is harmful to themselves or others. It can be very difficult for these young people to let go of their guilty feelings. But, being aware of where these feelings come from can help. People can and do learn to work past their guilt.

A Few Final Words

You're growing up, and growing up isn't always an easy thing to do, but it's important to remember that growing up has its more positive sides. We are becoming sexual beings as we move through puberty and into adulthood. Sexuality is a rich and meaningful part of our lives, a source of deep joy and contentment, and puberty, despite the problems it may present, is an exciting time in our lives. It is a time of many "firsts"— first period, first date, first kiss, first love, first job, first driver's license. It is a time when we begin to become our very own independent selves. We hope that this book has helped you to understand your puberty and to enjoy it all the more.

FOR FURTHER READING

BOOKS FOR YOUNG CHILDREN

Ideally sex education should begin at a very early age. One way to introduce the topic is through some of the excellent picture books for young children. The following are among our favorites and are appropriate for four- to eight-year-olds.

Dragonwagon, Crescent. *Windrose* (New York: Harper & Row, 1976). A lovely, lyrical picture book in which a mother describes to her child how the child was conceived and how it felt to carry the child and give birth.

Sheffield, Margaret. *Where Do Babies Come From?* (New York: Knopf, 1978).
This book explains puberty, sex, conception, pregnancy, and birth in terms that even a very young child can understand. It is sensitively done and beautifully illustrated.

Waxman, Stephanie. *What Is a Girl? What Is a Boy?* (Los Angeles: Peace Press, 1976).
This frank and forthright book, illustrated with nude photos of infants, children, and adults, deals with the physical differences between the two sexes.

BOOKS FOR OLDER READERS

Alyson, Sasha. *Young, Gay & Proud* (Boston: Alyson Publications, 1980).

A young person's guide to what it means to be gay; considered by many to be the best answer book for young gay people.

Bell, Ruth. *Changing Bodies, Changing Lives: A Book for Teens on Sex and Relationships* (New York: Random House, 1981).

A fine book, representing many points of view through quotes from teenagers themselves. The section on teenage pregnancy is especially good, and the one on mental health, depression, and suicide is outstanding. The book is geared toward the fifteen- to nineteen-year-old age group, but it could be valuable for younger and older people as well.

Betancourt, Jean. *Am I Normal?* (New York: Avon Books, 1983).

This book has lots of photos and tells the story of a thirteen-year-old boy who's going through puberty and is trying to be "cool" about it—but he wonders whether or not what's happening to him is normal.

Betancourt, Jean. *Dear Diary* (New York: Avon Books, 1983).

This book tells the story of a thirteen-year-old girl whose girlfriends are acting like there's something wrong with her because she hasn't gotten her period and doesn't have a boyfriend yet. She finally does, and she also gets answers to her questions about this whole business of growing up.

Calderone, Mary S., M.D. and Johnson, Eric W. *The Family Book About Sexuality,* rev. ed. (New York: Bantam Books, 1983).

Designed for the whole family, this book talks about how sexuality begins when we are only tiny babies, and how it develops through puberty and adulthood, and even into old age.

Comfort, Alex and Jane. *The Facts of Love: Living, Loving, and Growing* (New York: Crown, 1979).

This book covers many of the same topics dealt with in *Changing Bodies, Changing Lives,* but it is aimed at younger adolescents. More conservative parents may be more comfortable with this book than with the much franker presentation in Changing Bodies.

The Diagram Group. *Woman's Body: An Owner's Manual* and *Man's Body: An Owner's Manual* (New York: Bantam Books, 1977).
   Excellent books that have chapters on the sex organs and sexuality. They also cover other parts of the body, illness, body care, fitness, nutrition, and a lot more.

Gardner-Loulan, Joann; Lopez, Bonnie; and Quackenbush, Maria. *Period* (San Francisco: Volcano press, 1981).
   This excellent picture book deals with menstruation and is especially useful for introducing preteens to the topic. The illustrations feature all ethnic groups and even handicapped kids (which most books don't).

Madaras, Lynda and Area. *Lynda Madaras' Growing-Up Guide for Girls* (New York: Newmarket Press, 1986).
   Combines information about changing bodies during puberty with quizzes, checklists, drawings, and many personal stories about what it feels like to be growing up.

Madaras, Lynda and Saavedra, Dane. *The What's Happening to My Body? Book for Boys* (New York: Newmarket Press, 1984).
   This is a book that a teenage friend and I wrote for boys about puberty. Needless to say, we think it's a pretty good one. Although it was written for boys, many girls and parents have read it and told us they learned a lot from it.

Planned Parenthood. *Kids Need to Know.*
   Kids Need to Know is an information kit for parents and teens that includes booklets and pamphlets on topics such as sexuality and birth control. The kit is available from the Information and Education Department, Planned Parenthood, 1920 Marengo Street, Los Angeles, California 90033.

INFORMATION ABOUT AIDS

Madaras, Lynda. *Lynda Madaras Talks to Teens about AIDS* (New York: Newmarket Press, 1988).

Designed for teens aged fifteen through nineteen, many of whom may already be sexually active. Includes straightforward information on methods of transmission, high risk groups, and prevention through safe sex practices.

The National Public Health Service has a toll-free AIDS Hotline, 1-800-342-AIDS. In addition, there are some free pamphlets you can obtain by sending a self-addressed, stamped envelope to: AIDS and Children, Department of Health Education, New York University, 715 Broadway, New York, New York, 10003.

INDEX

(Page references in italics refer to illustrations.)

THE WHAT'S HAPPENING TO MY BODY? BOOK FOR GIRLS,
New Edition
A Growing-Up Guide for Parents and Daughters
Lynda Madaras with Area Madaras
Foreword by Cynthia Cooke, M.D.
288 pages; 44 drawings; bibliography; index.

THE WHAT'S HAPPENING TO MY BODY? BOOK FOR BOYS,
New Edition
A Growing-Up Guide for Parents and Sons
Lynda Madaras with Dane Saavedra
Foreword by Ralph I. Lopez, M.D.
272 pages; 34 drawings; bibliography; index.

Newly revised and updated, these two bestselling puberty education
books for 8- to 15-year-olds, their parents, and other concerned adults
now include information appropriate for this age level about AIDS,
other sexually transmitted diseases (STDs), and birth control.

THE WHAT'S HAPPENING? WORKBOOK FOR GIRLS
Lynda Madaras and Area Madaras
128 pages

The latest edition to Newmarket's parenting/teen-care library.
Quizzes, checklists, and innovative exercises encourage expression
of feelings about a young girl's changing body.

LYNDA MADARAS' GROWING-UP GUIDE FOR GIRLS
Lynda Madaras with Area Madaras
224 pages; 30 drawings; bibliography.

The companion workbook/journal to *The What's Happening to My
Body? Book for Girls* will help pre-teens and teens further explore
their changing bodies and their relationships with parents, teachers,
and friends; complete with space to record personal experiences.

LYNDA MADARAS TALKS TO TEENS ABOUT AIDS
An Essential Guide for Parents, Teachers, and Young People
Lynda Madaras
Foreword by Constance Wofsy, M.D.
128 pages; 9 drawings; resource guide; index.

Everything teens need to know to protect themselves against AIDS.
Written especially for 14- to 19-year olds (whether sexually active or
not), this book separates the facts from the rumors, explains the sexual
transmission of AIDS and its prevention (including comprehensive
information on abstinence and safe sex), and more.